Pediatric Endodontics

Anna B. Fuks • Benjamin Peretz
Editors

Pediatric Endodontics

Current Concepts in Pulp Therapy for Primary and Young Permanent Teeth

Springer

Editors
Anna B. Fuks
Department of Pediatric Dentistry
The Hebrew University Hadassah
School of Dental Medicine
Jerusalem
Israel

Benjamin Peretz
Department of Pediatric Dentistry
The Maurice and Gabriela Goldschleger
School of Dental Medicine
Tel Aviv University
Tel Aviv
Israel

ISBN 978-3-319-27551-2 ISBN 978-3-319-27553-6 (eBook)
DOI 10.1007/978-3-319-27553-6

Library of Congress Control Number: 2016933125

Springer Cham Heidelberg New York Dordrecht London

Printed on acid-free paper

Springer International Publishing AG Switzerland is part of Springer Science+Business Media (www.springer.com)

This book is dedicated to
Moises Fuks, my beloved husband and
long-term companion and friend
and to
Tamar, Neta and Alona Peretz, my beloved
and precious family

Anna B. Fuks and Benjamin Peretz

Preface

The initial idea for writing this book came because we felt that there has been an explosion of scientific knowledge on the understanding of the pulp tissue in the last two decades, which, in turn, affect the proper treatment for various pulp pathological conditions. This immense advancement has included the primary pulp also, and pediatric dentistry today, with regard to pulp treatment, can provide a better, more problem-oriented therapy and treatment to the affected primary pulp. Therefore, when we were approached by the Springer representative to write this book, we gladly agreed.

We felt that there was a need for students, undergraduate and postgraduate alike, as well as for the professional community to be familiarized with the current "state of the art" on pediatric endodontics. We made all efforts to cover the various aspects of the dentin-pulp complex in pediatric dentistry: from the understanding of biological concepts of the healthy pulp, through the pulp reactions to the deleterious effects of caries, to the various treatment modalities for each type of pulp injury, to the adverse reactions to various pulp dressing materials, and to the postoperative prognosis.

The better understanding of these topics led us to conclude that a conservative approach in the treatment of reversibly inflamed pulp needs to be emphasized. Thus, considerable attention has been given to the conservative approach to pulp treatment in primary and young permanent teeth. Our message stresses the paradigm shift toward conservative treatment modalities, relying on an accurate diagnosis based on signs and symptoms to assess the appropriateness of the technique for a specific case.

Notwithstanding, the traditional modes of treatment are also covered.

Understanding the new concepts regarding pulp treatment will guide practicing pediatric dentists and general dentists to select the proper mode of treatment.

A special emphasis has also been given to the future of pulp treatment, in light of the innovative knowledge on stem cells. At present, there is a consensus that the future of medicine and dentistry, particularly of pulp treatment, lies in the thorough research on stem cells.

We hope that this text will be useful to all students and dentists who treat children, to provide a better care for their teeth.

Jerusalem, Israel — Anna B. Fuks
Tel Aviv, Israel — Benjamin Peretz

Contents

Pediatric Endodontics: Past and Present Perspectives and Future Directions

1

Anna B. Fuks and Benjamin Peretz

Contents

Dentistry for children is one of the most needed of all specialties in dentistry. Yet, unawareness of newer concepts of present-day pediatric dentistry practice and the ultimate goals to be achieved still exist. The value of teaching pediatric dentistry cannot be overestimated as inadequate or unsatisfactory dental treatment during childhood may damage permanently the entire masticatory apparatus, leaving the individual with many of the dental problems so common in today's adult population [1].

The utmost goals of modern pediatric dentistry are to bring children into the permanent dentition after natural exfoliation of their healthy and/or properly treated primary teeth and instill a positive attitude toward keeping habits of optimal dental and oral health.

A.B. Fuks, DDS (✉)
Department of Pediatric Dentistry, The Hebrew University
Hadassah School of Dental Medicine, Jerusalem, 12272, Israel
e-mail: fuks@mail.huji.ac.il

B. Peretz, DMD
Department of Pediatric Dentistry, The Maurice and Gabriela
Goldschleger School of Dental Medicine, Tel Aviv, Israel
e-mail: bperetz@post.tau.ac.il

A.B. Fuks, B. Peretz (eds.), *Pediatric Endodontics: Current Concepts in Pulp Therapy for Primary and Young Permanent Teeth*,
DOI 10.1007/978-3-319-27553-6_1

1.1 Pediatric Endodontics

Pediatric dentistry is a unique specialty that deals with the total and comprehensive oral health care of children. As such, it involves all aspects of oral care ranging from prevention to restorative treatments. Historically, pediatric dentistry has evolved from an extraction-oriented practice at the beginning, where primary teeth with inflamed pulps were mostly extracted, and no focus has been put on preserving the pulp, to a specialty based on emphasizing prevention of oral and dental diseases.

A more conservative approach has been developed during the last decades regarding dental caries and specific modes of treatment such as minimal invasive dentistry and an increase use of prevention materials (mainly containing fluoride). This approach has been attributed to both developed diagnostic criteria and tools and to the new dental products and materials in the market. This approach goes further with regard to pulp therapy. It has long been established that the human dental pulp has a remarkable potential for self-healing when encountering a severe insult, especially in young patients, mainly due to the high degree of cellularity and vascularity. Incomplete caries removal, stepwise excavation, and indirect pulp treatment have been proposed to treat reversibly inflamed pulps. In addition, several techniques for managing irreversibly inflamed or necrotic pulps have been introduced in pediatric dentistry practice. Exposure of the pulp may occasionally be due to caries but may also occur by accident during cavity preparation or by fracture of the crown of the permanent maxillary incisors in particular.

Despite the extensive progress that has been achieved in prevention of dental caries worldwide, and the variety of treatment modalities to treat inflamed and/or infected pulp, a remarkable number of complications of untreated or poorly treated primary teeth and/or young immature permanent teeth are still encountered. This demands exact diagnosis, thorough knowledge of pulpal conditions and therapies, and also the value of the individual tooth for the occlusal development. Hence, pediatric endodontics has its own characteristics and includes the pulpal treatment of primary and young immature permanent teeth. It must always be seen in the total context of the dentition and the patient.

A review of the anatomy of primary teeth readily explains the frequent need for pulp therapy in these teeth. Specifically, Finn [1] and Ash [2] described twelve basic differences between primary and permanent teeth that can be summarized as follows: the enamel is thinner on primary teeth than on permanent teeth, and the thickness of the dentin between the pulp chambers and the enamel in primary teeth is less than in permanent teeth. The pulp, therefore, is correspondingly closer to the outer surface, and dental caries can progress and penetrate into the dentin more rapidly, leaving the tooth more susceptible to infection. Thus, pulp exposures caused by caries occur more frequently in primary teeth. If infection spreads to the alveolar bone, the developing permanent tooth may also be affected.

Pulp treatment of young permanent teeth must take into consideration the life expectancy of the young patient and provide the best conditions for the roots to develop and mature.

The practitioner should be familiar with the different treatment approaches to be able to select the most appropriate modality for each specific clinical situation.

1.2 Historical Perspective

The first method of capping exposed pulps was described by Phillip Pfaff, a dentist at the court of the Prussian King Friedrich II in Berlin in 1756 who used gold foils [3]. Several agents for direct pulp capping have been recommended ever since. The assumption that the pulp tissue must be irritated by cauterization in order to heal prevailed until the end of the nineteenth century, and most materials were used empirically. At the beginning of the twentieth century, it became obvious that microorganisms were the reason for pulp inflammation, and more attention was drawn to disinfecting agents that, although effective, were very cytotoxic. The lack of proper tools for achieving accurate diagnoses led to insufficient assessment of the pulp status leading to incorrect treatment selection. Thus, due to this fact, necrotic pulps were sometimes capped [3].

The first scientific clinical study to compare different capping materials was made by Dätwyler in 1921, whereupon zinc oxide-eugenol showed the best results. One year later, Rebel performed the first animal experiments with disastrous results, so he regarded the exposed pulp as a doomed organ. In 1920, Hermann introduced calcium hydroxide for root canal fillings. Between 1928 and 1930 he studied the reaction of vital pulp tissue to calcium hydroxide to prove that it was a biocompatible material. Since then, calcium hydroxide has been recommended by several authors for direct pulp capping, but it was only in the middle of the twentieth century was it regarded as the standard of care [3].

A Shift in the Paradigm of Treating Pulpally Involved Teeth

A change in clinical approach to pulpally involved teeth in pediatric patients will be proposed in this book and will be described in the different chapters. The change in approach involves a shift in the traditional paradigm regarding reversibly inflamed pulp from an "aggressive" approach involving total excavation of the carious dentin and the danger of exposing the pulp, towards a more "conservative" approach in which caries may be left in the pulpal wall to prevent pulp exposure. This approach is being slowly spread in the dental profession, and may become the treatment of choice for deep caries in modern pediatric dentistry practice.

As long as minimal invasive dentistry is still reluctantly accepted by the professional community many teeth with reversible pulp inflammation, that could otherwise be conservatively treated, will become pulpally involved. These teeth will be treated by the different pulp treatment modalities that will be described in this book.

1.3 The Scope of the Book

The nine chapters of this book will describe in detail the developmental and biomedical aspects of the primary pulp and comprehensive clinical diagnosis of the pulp leading to conservative approaches of pulp therapy, including stepwise excavation, indirect pulp treatment (IPT), and direct pulp capping. In the chapter on stepwise excavation and IPT, the Hall technique is mentioned. This technique, which includes cementation of a stainless steel crown on primary teeth without any caries removal or tooth preparation, has been shown to be successful in several clinical studies [4]. As this technique contradicts all established accepted principles of good clinical practice and it is still unknown what is the long-term effect on the development of the occlusion, the Hall technique is definitely a proof that after an accurate diagnosis, caries can be left on a tooth if properly sealed.

Furthermore, even though our message emphasizes the shift toward conservative approaches, these rely on an accurate diagnosis based on signs and symptoms to check the appropriateness of the technique for a specific case. Evidently, a thorough radiographic evaluation is essential for proper diagnosis. Thus, when a conservative approach is not indicated, the pulpotomy technique, as old as it is (over 40 years), will be presented, and the various dressing materials will be critically discussed. In addition, the nature of successful treatment and, more importantly, failures will be described.

Following the chapter on pulpotomy, an extensive and detailed chapter on pulpectomy and root canal filling (RCT) will be presented, describing in detail the rationale behind RCT, the techniques to perform RCT, the instruments, and the associated materials. Again, the success and failure rates of RCT will be described.

A special chapter will be dedicated to the importance of appropriate restorations of pulpally treated teeth, emphasizing the need of leakage prevention to improve the final prognosis.

Although this book is mainly dedicated to primary teeth, as previously mentioned, children often present pulp pathology in their immature permanent teeth. These teeth deserve a different treatment approach than the permanent teeth in adults, and for this reason, a special chapter dealing with this subject is included.

Finally, innovative experimental biological treatment modalities such as using stem cells, a new and developing area in medicine and in dentistry, will be presented. This approach will no doubt be one of the most prevailing treatment modalities in the future. It will expand the scope of conservative treatments, giving the clinician a more versatile arsenal of tools to deal with the damaged pulp.

1.4 The Aim of the Book

This book is aimed to familiarize dental students as well as general practitioners and pediatric dentists with the different treatment modalities and complications of uncontrolled caries, offering them the tools to diagnose the degree of pulp inflammation and thus select the most appropriate treatment.

This book is meant to be a tribute to Dr. Sidney B. Finn, one of the pioneers in pediatric dentistry and mentor of one of the editors (ABF). Dr. Finn's nice and warm personality, showing always a humane and empathic attitude toward the patients and parents, had a tremendous influence on Dr. Fuks's education and professional formation.

References

1. Finn SB. The children's dentist, his practice and his community. In: Finn SB, editor. Clinical Pedodontics. 4th ed. Clinical Pedodontics, Philadelphia: WB Saunders; 1973.
2. Ash M. Wheeler's dental anatomy, physiology and occlusion. 7th ed. Philadelphia: WB Saunders; 1992.
3. Dammaschke T. The history of direct pulp capping. J Hist Dent. 2008;56(1):9–23.
4. Innes NP, Stewart M. The hall technique, a simplified method for placing stainless steel crowns on primary molars, may be as successful as traditionally placed crowns. J Evid Based Dent Pract. 2015;15(2):70–2.

The Primary Pulp: Developmental and Biomedical Background

2

Anna B. Fuks, Josimeri Hebling, and Carlos Alberto de Souza Costa

Contents

A.B. Fuks, DDS (✉)
Department of Pediatric Dentistry, The Hebrew University Hadassah School of Dental Medicine, Jerusalem, 12272, Israel
e-mail: fuks@mail.huji.ac.il

J. Hebling, DDS, MS, PhD
Department of Orthodontics and Pediatric Dentistry, University Estadual Paulista – UNESP, Araraquara School of Dentistry, Rua Humaitá, 1.680 – Centro, Araraquara, SP 14.801-903, Brazil
e-mail: jhebling@foar.unesp.br

C.A. de Souza Costa, DDS, MS, PhD
Department of Physiology and Pathology, University Estadual Paulista – UNESP, Araraquara School of Dentistry, Rua Humaitá, 1.680 – Centro, Araraquara, SP 14.801-903, Brazil
e-mail: casouzac@foar.unesp.br

A.B. Fuks, B. Peretz (eds.), *Pediatric Endodontics: Current Concepts in Pulp Therapy for Primary and Young Permanent Teeth*,
DOI 10.1007/978-3-319-27553-6_2

2.1 Introduction

Maintaining the integrity and health of the oral tissues is the primary objective of pulp treatment. Premature loss of primary teeth can lead to malocclusion and/or to esthetic, phonetic, or functional problems. It is important to attempt to preserve pulp vitality whenever possible; however, when this is not feasible, the pulp can be entirely extirpated without significantly compromising the function of the tooth [1, 2].

For more than one century, several conservative pulp therapies have been employed empirically, with no scientific evidence. From the early 1970s, several clinical and laboratory studies started to appear in the literature, leading to the development of therapeutic methods based on experimental techniques [3].

Tziafas [4] reported that the current knowledge concerning the molecular and cellular mechanisms that take place during tooth development stresses the similarities between the developmental and regenerative tissue events. The author suggested that the most important challenge in dentistry during the last two decades has been how to integrate the current concepts of biomedical research into the problem of preservation of tooth structure and function during dental treatment. He also claimed that the present knowledge of the biological mechanisms of tooth development and regeneration can provide opportunities to design new strategies or agents for the preservation of tooth structures and functions.

Since the pulp of a primary tooth is histologically similar to that of a permanent tooth, the purpose of this chapter is to familiarize the reader with the characteristics of the development, structure, and function of the dentin–pulp complex. This knowledge will serve as a basis for discussing the diagnosis of pulp pathologies and the healing potential of the dentin–pulp complex against different noxious stimuli, which will be discussed in future chapters.

2.2 Formation of the Dentin–Pulp Complex

The dental pulp is a specialized connective tissue of mesenchymal origin surrounded by tubular dentin walls occupying the pulp chamber and the root canal.

The specific group of pulp cells, known as odontoblasts, is responsible for the synthesis and deposition of the collagen-rich dentin organic matrix, which is further mineralized around the pulp tissue. Therefore, dentin and the pulp remain closely associated during development and throughout life and are commonly referred to as the dentin–pulp complex (Fig. 2.1a, b).

Events that take place on the dentin reverberate to the pulp and vice versa [5].

The dentin–pulp complex is surrounded on the crown by dental enamel and on the root by cementum, periodontal ligament, and bone. The harmony of the complex is impaired if the surrounding tissues suffer some kind of injury that can reach the pulp by the root canal or through the dentinal tubules [5].

Although the tooth is a unique organ, the principles that guide its development are shared in common with other organs such as lung, kidney, heart, mammary

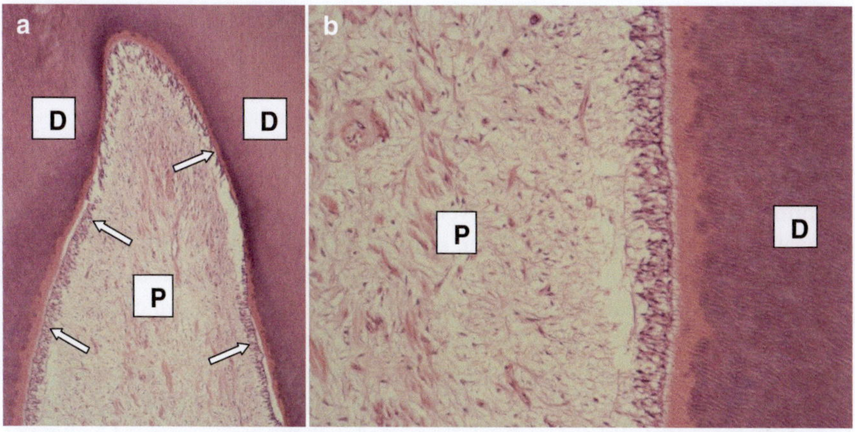

Fig. 2.1 (**a**) Histological section obtained from sound primary teeth. The tubular dentin (*D*) was synthesized and deposited by the odontoblasts (*arrows*), which are organized in a defined layer of cells that remains underlying this mineralized tissue. H/E, 32× (*P* Pulp). (**b**) High magnification of the (**a**). Note the continuous layer of odontoblasts beneath the thin layer of predentin. The subjacent pulp tissue (*P*) exhibits a number of cells, capillaries, and a loose extracellular matrix. H/E, 160× (*D* dentin)

glands, and hair follicles [6]. The most important developmental events are those guiding epithelial–mesenchymal interactions, which are characterized by a molecular cross talk between two tissues of different origins, the ectoderm and the mesenchyme [6].

Different stages of tooth development have been recognized at a microscopic level by their histologic appearance and were classically described as the dental lamina, bud, cap, and the early and late bell stages. In the modern literature, a functional terminology has been used to describe odontogenesis into four phases: initiation, morphogenesis, cell differentiation (cytodifferentiation), and matrix apposition [6]. The dental lamina is the first sign of tooth development. At the *lamina stage*, cells of the dental epithelium and those of the underlying ectomesenchyme divide at different rates and continue to grow and thicken to form a bud [6]. At the *bud stage*, cells of the ectomesenchyme proliferate and condense to give rise to the dental papilla. These cells have increased ability to proliferate, mobilize, and differentiate.

The *morphogenetic phase* involves the stages of bud, cap, and initial bell phase. During this period, a number of ectomesenchymal cells adjacent to the epithelium increase inside the ectomesenchyme, producing the site of origin of the dental papilla and of the dental follicle. These will develop into the dentin–pulp complex and into the support tissues of the tooth, respectively [6]. The formation of the enamel knot, during the transition from bud to cap, marks the beginning of crown formation. The cells of the enamel knot do not grow and serve as a signal for the cuspid formation pattern, influencing the form of the crown and the development of the dental papilla [6].

During the initial bell phase, the epithelium cells assume different morphologies, giving rise to the enamel organ, also called dental organ. This enamel organ is composed of the following four different stratums: internal enamel epithelium, stratum intermedium, stellate reticulum, and external enamel epithelium.

The internal epithelium of the enamel organ interacts with the undifferentiated superficial mesenchymal cells (also known as embryonic cells) of the dental papilla to form enamel, dentin, and pulp. Overall, cells of the internal dental epithelium elongate and become highly columnar, starting the late bell stage (*phase of cytodifferentiation*). This modification of the internal dental epithelium cells serves as a signal for the peripheral mesenchymal cells of the dental papilla, which after lining the basement membrane differentiate and assume an elongated morphology with odontoblast phenotype [6]. This phenomenon, characterized as differentiation of odontoblasts, has been intensely studied, leading to important advances in the knowledge of pulpal biology, particularly related with the mechanisms of healing of this specialized connective tissue against injuries and different pathological stimuli. More details about this issue will be discussed later in this chapter.

It is important to know the basic process of differentiation of the superficial undifferentiated mesenchymal cells from the dental papilla by stimuli expressed by cells of the internal dental epithelium. Growth factors, particularly those belonging to the superfamily TGF-β, are expressed by these epithelial cells. While the mesenchymal cells of the most superficial region of the dental papilla become competent, the last mitosis of the mother cell is positioned adjacent to the basal membrane. The daughter cells remain in the internal area of the papilla and will be part of the cell-rich zone that is clearly observed in the mature pulp. At this point both mother and daughter cells are referred as pre-odontoblasts because they assume the competency to differentiate into odontoblasts. Between the internal dental epithelium cells and the pre-odontoblasts is the basal membrane, which is composed of collagen, laminin, heparin sulfate, and other proteoglycans.

This basal membrane has an important role in the reciprocal activation of the epithelium/mesenchyme, resulting in a variety of epigenetic interactions, determining the phenotype of the odontoblasts. After the epithelial cells secrete the growth factors of the TGF-β superfamily, these bioactive proteins remain attached to the basal membrane. The components of the basal membrane activate these TGFs to interact with membrane receptors of the pre-odontoblasts. The translation of these signals results in the activation of the pre-odontoblasts, which start to secrete more growth factors and express the *msxs* genes. The final differentiation of the pre-odontoblasts into odontoblasts occurs only after the interaction of the fibronectin, which is deposited on the basal membrane and the 165 KDa pre-odontoblasts membrane receptors. The sequence of differentiation of the dental papilla mesenchymal cells into odontoblasts until the beginning of the synthesis and deposition of collagen-rich dentinal matrix is presented in Fig. 2.2.

The odontoblasts synthesize the dentinal organic matrix both adjacent to the cellular body and close to the mineralization *fronts*. During the period of upregulation of the TGFs, the pre-odontoblasts start to synthesize fibronectin and express the membrane protein 165 KDa, which is required to interact with the fibronectin.

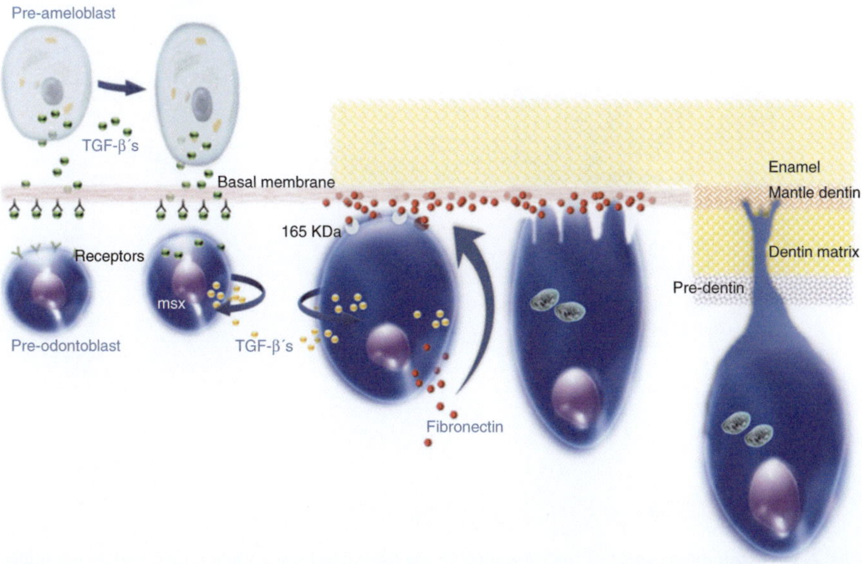

Fig. 2.2 Mechanism by which the pulpal mesenchymal cells present in the periphery of the dental papilla are differentiated into odontoblasts (Adapted from [31]) (J. Hebling, 2015)

The *msxs* homeoproteins are probably involved in the reorganization of the pre-odontoblast cytoskeleton, which plays an important role in the process of differentiating into elongated cells, referred to as odontoblasts.

The mineralization process is mainly dependent on the odontoblasts' activities: they release phospholipids and alkaline phosphatase containing vesicles that produce the hydroxyapatite crystals. The dentin matrix mineralization is heterogeneous, by globular calcification, resulting in *fronts* of mineralization or calcospherites. With continuous growth, the crystals tend to fuse (secondary mineralization), forming a mineralized mass around the odontoblastic processes, granting the dentin a tubular aspect (system of dentinal tubules). The portion of the dental papilla that is involved with dentin becomes the dental pulp. The odontoblasts form the dentin, but depend on it to become the pulp. The direction of the odontoblasts is towards the center, in relation to the dental pulp, and the decrease of the internal space favors a curved path of these cells. Once the first layer of dentin is formed, the cells of the internal epithelium (pre-ameloblasts) elongate and differentiate into ameloblasts starting to produce the enamel organic matrix, which becomes mineralized almost instantaneously.

As dentin is formed, the most cervical cells of the internal epithelium of the enamel organ become pre-ameloblasts, an event that occurs from the incisal (or from the cuspids) to the cervical area. When the dentin formation approximates the cervical loop, the cells of internal and external epithelium of the enamel organ proliferate from the loop, forming a double layer of cells, also known as Hertwig's epithelial root sheath. The expansion of the sheath is followed by the formation of the radicular dentin. The cells of the dental follicle closer to the external layer of the

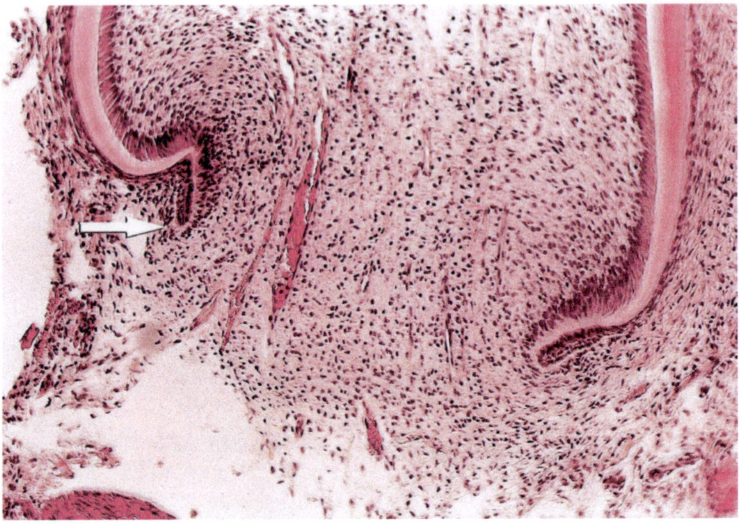

Fig. 2.3 Histological aspect of the formation of the apex. Hertwig's sheath, involved by ectomesenchymal cells of the papilla, can be seen on the left (Courtesy Prof. Roberto Holland, 2008)

sheath differentiate into cementoblasts and start to produce the cementum organic matrix; the follicle also produces the periodontal ligament and alveolar bone. There is a free border on the epithelial sheath, the epithelial diaphragm, which closes slowly as the root is formed (Fig. 2.3). As long as the apex of the root is not totally formed, there will be dental papilla, composed of ectomesenchymal cells. This has clinical relevance, because part of these cells can remain vital even after pulp necrosis. In this specific condition, it is possible to have a continuous apexogenesis or the formation of the radicular apex with dentin. When there is a severe reduction in the number of ectomesenchymal cells in the dental papillae, the tooth can still have apexification induced by an intracanal dressing [5]. This issue will be dealt in detail in Chap. 8.

2.3 The Dental Pulp

The dental pulp is a specialized connective tissue confined between rigid walls of mineralized tissues (dentin, enamel, and cementum). The dental pulp can communicate with the external environment of the tooth through the apical foramen, foramina, and/or lateral canals providing the pulp with a low-tolerance environment, because the nutritional substrate comes from the vascularization that passes through the small foramens and foramina.

Loose connective tissue forms the stroma (nutritional supportive tissue) and the parenchyma (functional tissue) of several organs of the human body. In the pulp, this loose connective tissue forms both the stroma and the parenchyma at the same time, as it sustains itself and the dentin substrate and produces dentin. With the

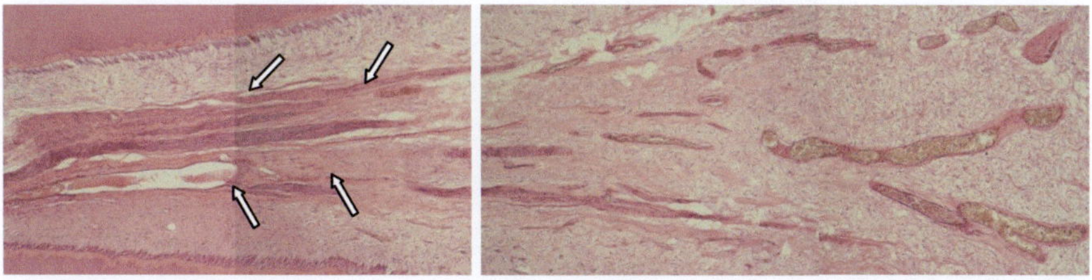

Fig. 2.4 Sections obtained from human sound teeth showing the radicular (*left*) and coronal (*right*) portions of the pulp tissue. Note the fibrous connective pulp tissue with vascular–nervous sheath close to the apical foramen (*arrows*). Conversely, the coronal pulp exhibits loose connective tissue with a number of blood vessels. H/E, 32×

production of dentin, the pulp remains enclosed within the central part of the tooth, having a coronal and a radicular portion. In uni-radicular teeth, the coronal and radicular pulp tissues are contiguous, but in multi-radicular teeth, the floor of the pulp chamber has a clear distinction: the coronal pulp is rich in cells and extracellular matrix, while the radicular pulp has more fibers, and the vascular–nervous sheath is more concentrated, with less anastomosis (Fig. 2.4).

2.3.1 Odontoblasts

The odontoblasts have been traditionally described as cells lining the periphery of the pulpal space and extending their cytoplasmic processes into the dentinal tubules. These cells have several junctions, which allow for intercellular communication and help to maintain the relative position of one cell to another. In young permanent teeth, the pulp tissue exhibits defined zones. The cell-free zone is located just below the odontoblastic layer and contains an extensive plexus of unmyelinated nerves and blood capillaries. The cell-rich zone, which presents a number of undifferentiated mesenchymal cells, is observed adjacent to the cell-free zone. The core of the dental pulp contains larger blood vessels and nerves, which are surrounded by large area of extracellular matrix. This pulp morphology is similar to that observed in primary teeth, but the zones are not so well defined (Fig. 2.5a, b).

Although this description is correct during active dentinogenesis, it is now accepted that the size of the odontoblasts and the content of their cytoplasmic organelles vary throughout their life cycle and are closely related to their functional activity. The relationship between the size of the odontoblasts and their secretory activity can be demonstrated by differences in their size in the crown and in the root, and different dentinogenic rates may be expressed in these two areas of the tooth [7].

The odontoblasts are highly specialized cells and are responsible for the formation of dentin. Due to the extension of their cytoplasmic processes into the dentinal tubules, these cells compose the main part of the dentin–pulp complex. When this complex is damaged by disease or attrition, or is affected by operative procedures, it reacts in an attempt to defend the pulp tissue.

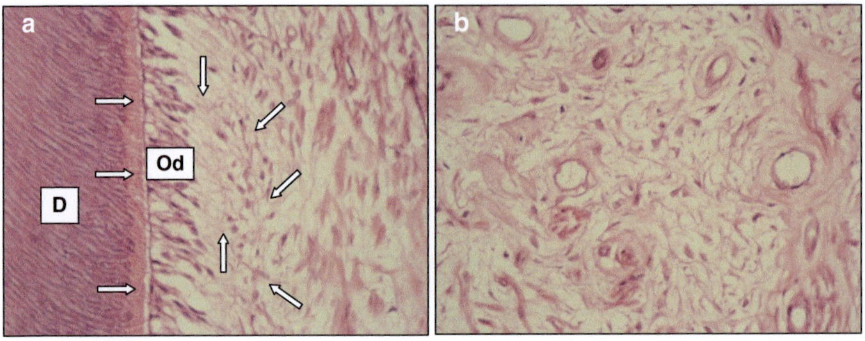

Fig. 2.5 (**a**) Sections obtained from human sound primary teeth. Note the presence of tubular dentin (*D*), predentin (*horizontal arrows*), odontoblast layer (*Od*), cell-free zone (*vertical arrows*), cell-rich zone (*oblique arrows*), and the core of the pulp. H/E, 160×. (**b**) The core of the pulp tissue contains a number of blood vessels and nerves, which are surrounded by a large area of extracellular matrix. H/E, 160×

2.4 Dentin Structure and Composition

Dentin is the most abundant mineral component of the teeth. It is composed of 70 % inorganic crystals (hydroxyapatite), 20 % collagen fibers and other proteins, and 10 % water (all by %volume). Dentin can be classified as *primary*, *secondary*, *or tertiary*, according to the time of development and the histological characteristics of the tissue.

2.4.1 Types of Dentin

The *primary dentin* is composed by the mantle dentin and by the circumpulpal dentin, which are physiological structures deposited up to the eruption of the tooth and its contact with the antagonist. Mantle dentin is the first dentin to be formed. It is deposited along the enamel–dentin or dentin–cementum junction, parallel to the tissues coating it. It is almost totally free of developmental defects. The odontoblasts, when supported by the basal membrane, have several cytoplasmic projections. This results in mantle dentin that is highly branched on the periphery converging into a single prolongation towards the center of the pulp chamber. Mantle dentin has an approximate thickness of 80–100 μm. The circumpulpal dentin is formed after the deposition of the mantle dentin and constitutes the majority of the dentin. Since the odontoblasts produce the organic dentin matrix centripetally concerning the pulp, the space available becomes increasingly reduced leading to an "S"-shaped curvature in the circumpulpal dentin, which is more pronounced at the crown and more discrete at the root [5].

Secondary dentin is also a physiological structure formed after the radicular dentin, maintaining the tubular pattern of the circumpulpal dentin, but its formation is slower and less regular. It is deposited more on the roof and the floor of the pulp

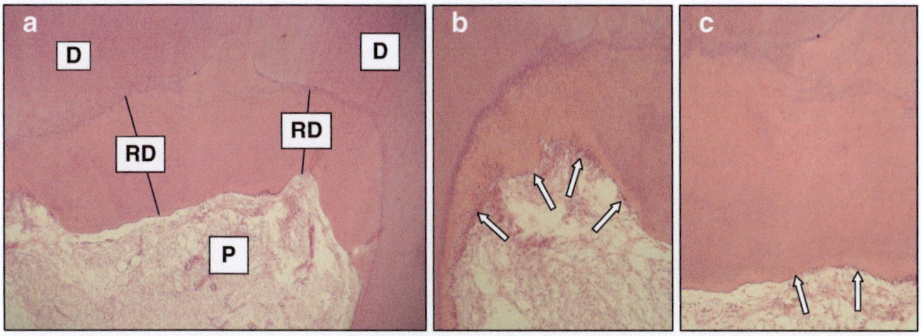

Fig. 2.6 (**a**) Section obtained from primary teeth with chronic occlusal caries (slight stimulus). Note the thick layer of tubular reactionary dentin (*RD*) deposited in the upper area of the pulp horn (*P*). (*D*) represents dentin. H/E, 32×. (**b**, **c**) High magnifications of (**a**). Note the tubular dentin deposited by primary odontoblasts (*arrows*) subjected to a low-intensity stimulus (chronic caries). H/E, 64×

chamber, reducing the pulp horns and the pulpal chamber asymmetrically. Approximately 1–1.5 μm of dentin matrix is incrementally deposited per day inside the pulp chamber.

Tertiary dentin is not a physiological structure, since it is produced in response to stimuli from the external environment, such as caries, attrition, abrasion, restorative procedures, etc. The formation of tertiary dentin occurs adjacent to the stimuli, modifying the pulpal and dentinal architecture. This dentin can be *reactionary*, when produced by preexisting odontoblasts, or *reparative*, which occurs with the replacement of dead odontoblasts by new odontoblasts, termed as odontoblast-like cells.

When low-intensity stimuli are applied to the odontoblasts, they respond by moving rapidly and centripetally in relation to the pulp. These cells then deposit a matrix that contains irregular and convoluted tubules. The morphology of recently produced dentinal matrix is characterized by the continuity with the existing dentin and is known as reactionary dentin (Fig. 2.6a–c).

Conversely, when the injury to the odontoblasts is intense and some of them die, new odontoblasts are differentiated from pre-odontoblasts (mesenchymal cells that were formed during dentinogenesis and remained partially in the cell-rich zone of the adult pulp). These new odontoblasts deposit a matrix of heterogeneous dentin, which is known as reparative dentin (Fig. 2.7). The process of deposition of reparative dentin is more complex than that of reactionary dentin, because it occurs by differentiation of the pulpal cells. In this case, undifferentiated reserve mesenchymal cells are used to replace the odontoblasts during the performance of some operative procedures or even during the fast progression of an acute caries lesion. Consequently, the number of mesenchymal cells (stem cells) decreases in the pulp tissue, leading to a reduced potential of healing [8]. Thus, aggression to the dentin–pulpal complex should be prevented to maintain its functional nature and physiologic metabolism, preventing its fast aging.

The predentin is a thin layer of collagen-rich dentin matrix (about 20 μm thick) recently synthesized by the odontoblasts. As described previously, this non-mineralized dentin matrix presents *fronts* of mineralization, also known as

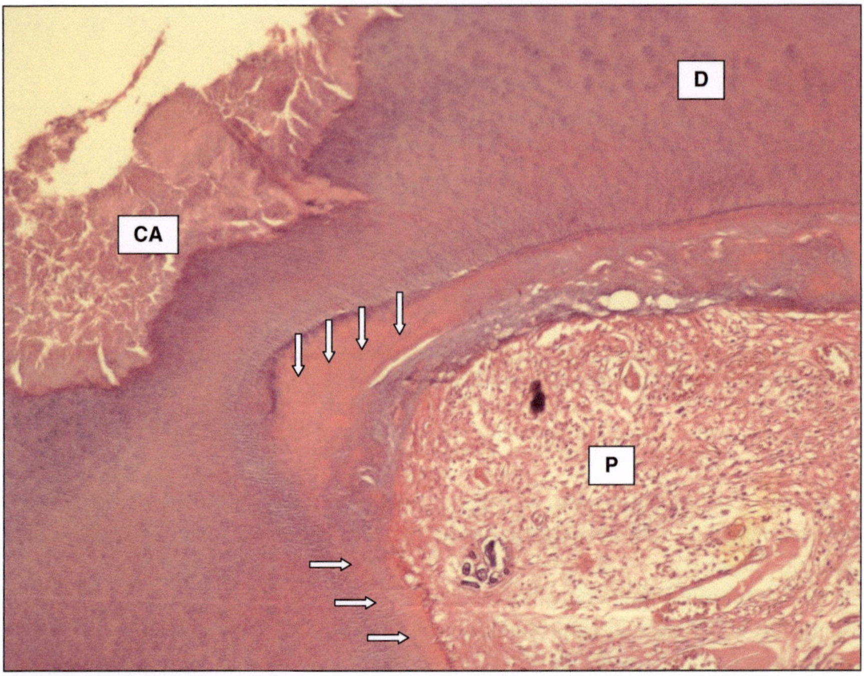

Fig. 2.7 Section obtained from primary teeth with acute occlusal caries (*CA*). Note the layer of tubular reactionary dentin (*horizontal arrows*) deposited in the lower part of the picture where the primary odontoblasts were far from the intense stimulus (pay attention to the dentinal tubule orientation). However, in the upper area of the picture, where the pulp is close to the very deep caries lesion (*CA*), a thick layer of reparative dentin with no tubules, termed as reparative dentin (*vertical arrows*), can be observed. H/E, 32× (*D* Dentin, *P* Pulp)

calcospherites (Fig. 2.8). Failure of the calcospherites to fuse leads to the formation of hypomineralized areas, known as interglobular dentin. These areas are more visible in the radicular dentin, where the dentin is produced simultaneously with the eruptive process, and on the most external portion of the coronal dentin, at the limit between the mantle and the circumpulpal dentin. Predentin consists mainly of types I and III collagen, glycoproteins, and proteoglycans.

Another type of hypocalcification is the Tomes' grainy layer that is formed by the terminal loops and branches of the odontoblastic membrane. This membrane configuration is developed during the formation of the radicular dentin, giving to the peripheral dentin a grainy appearance.

Dentin is composed of tubules. As the odontoblasts secrete the organic matrix, they emit a projection that is surrounded by liquid, providing the tubular aspect. The tubules have a lightly conical shape, due to the mineralization process of the peritubular dentin that occurs throughout the life of the tooth. The tubules extend through the entire thickness of the dentin, following the sinuous track of the odontoblasts. The number of dentinal tubules varies according to the area when different teeth are

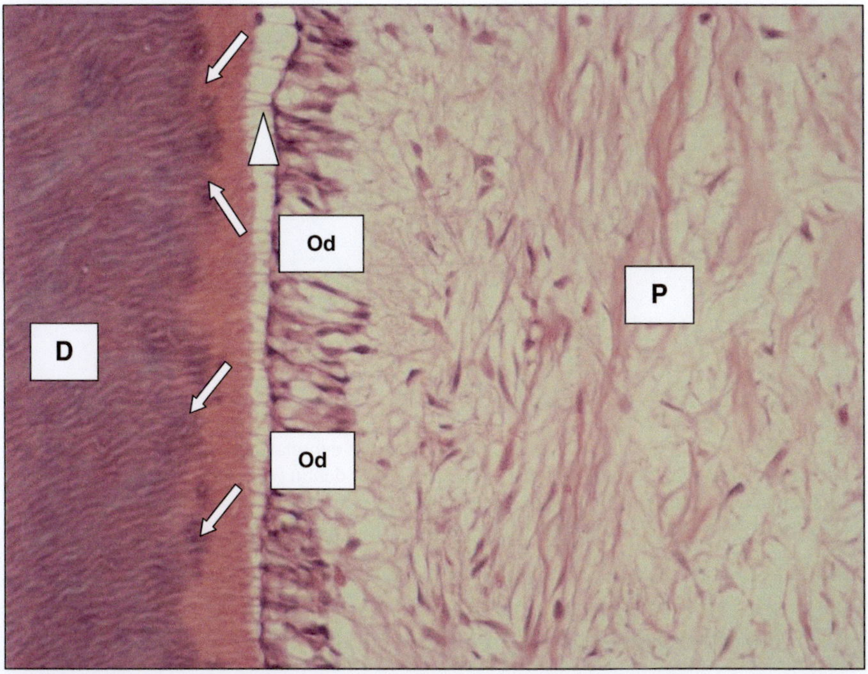

Fig. 2.8 Section obtained from sound primary teeth. Between the tubular dentin and the thin layer of predentin one can see the fronts of mineralization – calcospherites (*oblique arrows*). Note the odontoblasts (*Od*) with their cytoplasmic processes which get inside the dentinal tubules (*head arrow*) *D* dentin. *P* pulp. H/E, 125×

compared. It has been demonstrated that at the enamel–dentin junction (superficial dentin), there are approximately 20,000 tubules/mm^2, while near the predentin (deep dentin), this number increases to approximately 75,000 tubules/mm^2.

The dentin surrounding the periphery of the dentinal tubules is known as peritubular or intertubular dentin. Intertubular dentin is present between dentinal tubules. The odontoblast cytoplasmic processes remain within the dentinal tubules (Fig. 2.8).

Communications among the dentinal tubules, known as dentinal canaliculus, are frequently observed. The peritubular dentin that constitutes the walls of the dentinal tubules is four times harder than intertubular dentin, since it consists of approximately 96 % of hydroxyapatite crystals. Mild stimuli from the external environment, such as attrition and caries, may cause obliteration of the dentinal tubules, resulting in dentin sclerosis. Intertubular dentin is partially composed of collagen fibrils positioned perpendicularly to the long axis of the tubules, surrounding the tubules (Fig. 2.9a, b). The conditioning of the dentin substrate with acidic agents or chelating substances decreases or removes the peritubular dentin on the surface, leaving a mesh of intertubular collagen exposed to the action of bonding agents or to bacteria from decay [9, 10].

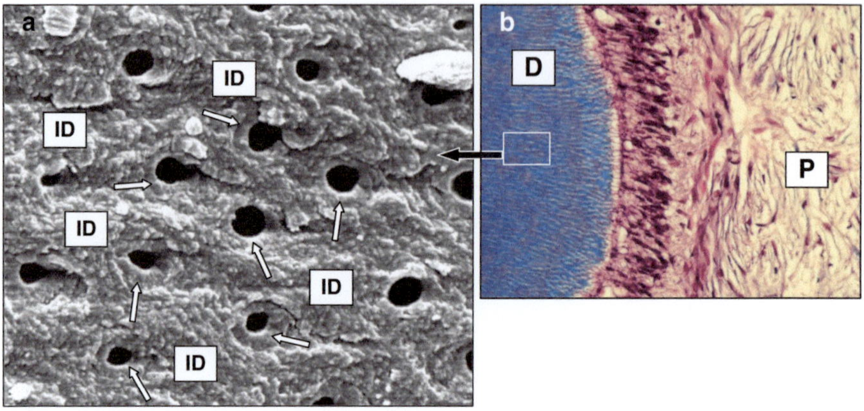

Fig. 2.9 (**a**) Morphology of the dentin structure. Note the dentinal tubules surrounded by peritubular dentin (*arrows*) as well as a large area of intertubular dentin (*ID*). MEV, 3.000×. (**b**) Dentin–pulp complex. *D* dentin. *P* pulp. Cytoplasmic processes from odontoblasts are observed inside the dentinal tubules. Masson's trichrome, 125×

2.5 Factors Affecting the Dentin–Pulp Complex Response to Stimuli in Primary Teeth

Although the life span of primary teeth is shorter and their dentin is thinner when compared to that of permanent teeth, the dentin–pulp complex response to dental caries in human primary teeth is similar to that of permanent teeth, including a reduction in the number of the odontoblasts and an increase in the number of inflammatory cells. These are found under very deep lesions and are less numerous in more distant regions, being almost absent in the radicular apical pulp [11]. The primary dentition is frequently subjected to stimuli such as trauma or caries with associated pulpal inflammation [12]. The same factors affect both the dentin–pulp responses in primary as well as permanent teeth, with respect to external stimuli.

2.6 The Deleterious Effects of Bacterial Infiltration at the Restorative Material Margins

A significant number of studies have implicated the presence of bacteria and their products as responsible for induction of the most severe forms of pulp inflammation. The role of bacteria in the inflammatory reaction was demonstrated by spontaneous healing of pulp exposures in germ-free animals [13] and subsequently by cavities restored with different materials and surface sealed with zinc oxide–eugenol cement to prevent any bacterial contamination originating from microleakage [14].

The presence of bacteria in cavities with a remaining dentin thickness (RDT) of less than 0.25 mm stimulates a more severe pulpal inflammatory reaction than in similar cavity preparations in the absence of bacteria [15]. Thus, the presence of bacteria always increases the mean grade of pulpal inflammation regardless of the RDT [16]. The presence of bacteria in class V cavity was also observed to result in a significant

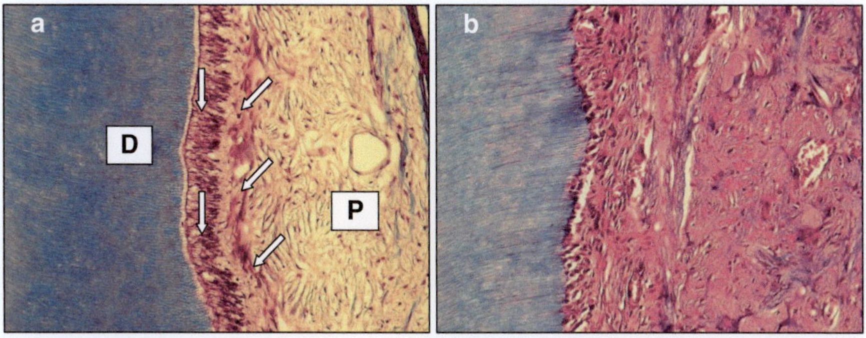

Fig. 2.10 (**a**) Section obtained from a young sound premolar in which a very deep class V cavity was prepared and the cavity floor lined with hard-setting calcium hydroxide cement. Note the pulp tissue with normal histological characteristics. Masson's trichrome, 64× (*D* Dentin, *P* Pulp; *vertical arrows* odontoblast layer; *oblique arrows* cell-rich zone). (**b**) In this human premolar, the cavity floor (dentin) was conditioned and a resin-based material was used as liner. Note the intense inflammatory response associated with complete pulp tissue disorganization. No microleakage at the cavity walls was observed after using a specific staining technique (Brown and Brenn) widely employed for disclosing bacteria. Masson's trichrome, 64×

decrease in the number of odontoblasts per unit area; this effect was more pronounced in deep cavities with RDT less than 0.5 mm than in cavities with RDT greater than 0.5 mm [16]. One can conclude that the ability to maintain an effective seal to protect the pulp from recurrent injury resulting from bacterial microleakage is a decisive factor in the clinical success of restorative products [17]. However, a number of studies performed in human teeth have shown pulpal inflammation in the absence of bacteria [8, 18–22], clearly indicating that other factors, such as the toxicity of dental material components capable of diffusing through dentinal tubules, are also responsible, at least in part, for pulp injury after restorative treatment (Fig. 2.10a, b).

2.7 The Protective Role of the Remaining Dentin Thickness (RDT)

It was found in an in vivo study that the cavity RDT is an important factor mediating pulpal inflammatory activity, particularly when the RDT is reduced to less than 0.3 mm [8, 22]. With an RDT less than 0.25 mm, a significant decrease in the number of odontoblasts was observed together with minimal reactionary dentin repair [23, 24]. It was recently demonstrated that very deep class V cavities prepared in human premolars (RDT thinner than 0.3 mm) which were subjected to adhesive restorations resulted in inflammatory pulp reaction associated with inner dentin resorption [8, 22, 25]. The presence of an RDT of more than 500 mm delays the diffusion of noxious materials into the dental pulp. In this clinical situation, the odontoblasts maintain their metabolism, or, in case of a slight stimulus, they may secrete a reactionary dentin, increasing the total distance between the restorative material and the pulp [8]. Any additional decrease in the dentin thickness to less than 500 mm results in a significant reduction in the number of odontoblasts.

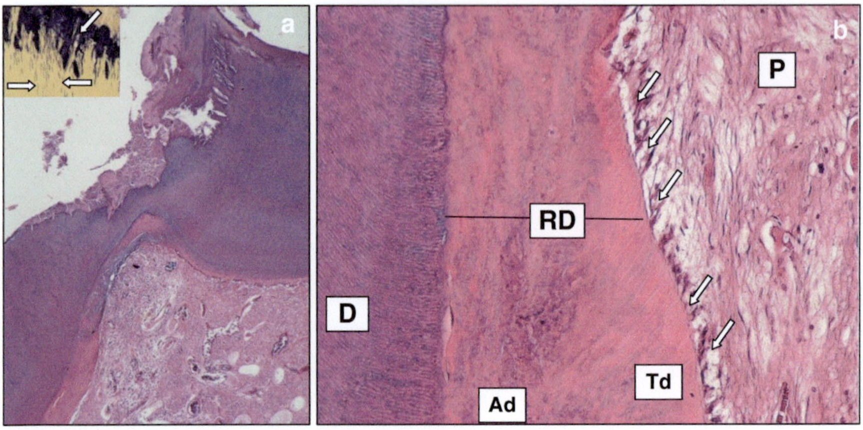

Fig. 2.11 (**a**) Deep carious lesion in primary first molar. H/E. 32×. The small image characterizes the necrotic dentin (*oblique arrow*) and the presence of microorganisms inside the dentinal tubules (*horizontal arrows*). Brown and Brenn technique, 125×. Note the intense inflammatory pulp reaction associated with complete tissue disorganization. (**b**) Detail of (**a**). Note the intense deposition of reparative dentin (*RD*) adjacent to the primary dentin (*D*). A heterogeneous and atubular dentin matrix (*Ad*) containing parts of dead odontoblasts as well as a tubular dentin (*Td*) deposited by the new odontoblast-like cells (*arrows*) can be observed. H/E, 125× (*P* Pulp)

This reduction may be compensated for by the differentiation of odontoblast-like cells from progenitor pulp cells, which migrate to the injury site and secrete reparative dentin. The reparative dentin decreases the dentin permeability and increases the distance between the restorative material and the pulp, protecting it from noxious products. However, in this specific condition, the number of mesenchymal stem cells decreases, interfering with the potential of pulpal healing in case of further damage to the dentin–pulp complex. Thus, the RDT appears to provide an important protective barrier against toxins, bacterial infiltration, or any noxious material applied to dentin. In this way, it seems adequate to protect the pulp tissue against irritant stimuli by using biocompatible materials as liners in very deep cavities [8].

Based on the remaining dentin thickness, three situations can be taken into consideration:

1. Initial carious lesion or shallow cavity preparations (RDT > 500 mm): a localized reactionary dentin may be secreted facing the restoration site, and intratubular mineralization (dentin sclerosis) occurs, resulting in a significant decrease in the dentin permeability and pulp protection. It has been suggested that this stimulation may be due to signaling molecules (i.e., TGF-b1, BMP-2 liberated from the dentin during demineralization) [26].
2. Carious lesion progression implying a deep cavity preparation (RDT < 500 mm): these lesions may lead to partial death of odontoblast. Depending on the pulp inflammatory intensity, progenitor/stem cells can migrate to the injury site and differentiate to give rise to a new generation of odontoblast-like cells. These cells are responsible for the deposition of a specific type of tertiary dentin termed as reparative dentin, as described above [27, 28] (Fig. 2.11a, b).

3. During a subsequent restorative process, deep cavity preparations with RDTs between 250 and 40 mm lead to poor tertiary dentin repair activity [15]. These result from impaired odontoblast dentin secretory activity due to cellular injury [29]. The study demonstrated that the mean number of intact odontoblasts found beneath this kind of cavity preparation was 36% lower than the number found beneath similar preparations with an RDT between 500 and 250 mm. This lack in the ability of the odontoblasts to provide adequate pulp repair and pulp protection after deep cavity preparation has been supported by observations of a persistent inflammatory pulpal response and odontoblast displacement following such deep cavity preparations [29].

2.8 Clinical Recommendations

In clinical situations, conservative careful cavity preparations should be carried out: intermittent cutting movement, air/spray cooling, and use of new burs. In addition, biocompatible, antibacterial, and bioactive dental products must be used as liners to protect the pulp tissue against toxic components released from restorative materials capable of diffusing across the dentin [20, 30].

References

1. Fuks AB. Pulp therapy in the primary and young permanent dentitions. Dent Clin North Am. 2000;44:571–96.
2. Fuks AB. Pulp therapy for the primary dentition. In: Pinkham JR, editor. Pediatric dentistry: infancy through adolescence. Philadelphia: Saunders; 2005.
3. Massara MLA, Toledo OA. Terapia endodontica em deciduos. In: Toledo OA, editor. Odontopediatria, fundamentos para a pratica clinica. 3rd ed. Sao Paulo, Brazil: Editorial Premier; 2005.
4. Tziafas D. Dentinogenic potential of the dental pulp: facts and hypotheses. Endod Top. 2010;17:42–64.
5. Costa CAS, Figueiredo JAP, Hebling J, Estrela C. Pulp biology. In: Estrela C, editors. Endodontic science, vol 1. Artes Medicas, Sao Paulo, Brazil; 2009.
6. D'Souza R. Development of the pulp–dentin complex. In: Hargreaves KM, Goodies HE, editors. Seltzer and Bender's dental pulp. Chicago: Quintessence Int; 2002.
7. Smith AJ. Dentin formation and repair. In: Hargreaves KM, Goodies HE, editors. Seltzer and Bender's dental pulp. Chicago: Quintessence Int; 2002.
8. de Souza Costa CA, Hebling J, Scheffel DL, Soares DG, Basso FG, Ribeiro AP. Methods to evaluate and strategies to improve the biocompatibility of dental materials and operative techniques. Dent Mater. 2014;30(7):769–84. doi:10.1016/j.dental.2014.04.010. Epub 2014 May 28.
9. Sardella TN, de Castro FL, Sanabe ME, Hebling J. Shortening of primary dentin etching time and its implication on bond strength. J Dent. 2005;33(5):355–62. Epub 2004 Dec 13.
10. Scheffel DL, Tenuta LM, Cury JA, Hebling J. Effect of acid etching time on demineralization of primary and permanent coronal dentin. Am J Dent. 2012;25(4):235–8.
11. Di Nicolo R, Guedes-Pinto AC, Carvalho YR. Histopathology of the pulp of primary molars with active and arrested dentinal caries. J Clin Pediatr Dent. 2000;25:47–9.
12. Klinge RF. Further observations on tertiary dentin in human deciduous teeth. Adv Dent Res. 2001;15:76–9.
13. Kakehashi S, Stanley HR, Fitzgerald RJ. The effect of surgical exposures of dental pulp in germ free and conventional laboratory rats. Oral Surg Oral Med Oral Pathol. 1965;20:340–9.

14. Cox CF, Keall CL, Keall HJ, Ostro E, Bergenholtz G. Biocompatibility of surface-sealed dental materials against exposed pulps. J Prosthet Dent. 1987;57:1–8.
15. Murray PE, About I, Tranquil JC, Recusant M, Smith AJ. Restorative pulpal and repair responses. J Am Dent Assoc. 2001;132:482–91.
16. About I, Murray PE, Franquin JC, Remusat MAJ. Pulpal inflammatory responses following non carious class V restorations. Oper Dent. 2001;26:336–42.
17. Qvist V. Correlation between marginal adaption of composite resin restorations and bacterial growth in cavities. Scand J Dent Res. 1980;88:296–300.
18. Qvist V, Staltze K, Qvist J. Human pulp reactions to resin restorations performed with different acid-etch restorative procedures. Acta Odontol Scand. 1989;47:253–63.
19. Costa CAS, Giro EM, do Nascimento AB, Teixeira HM, Hebling J. Short-term evaluation of the pulpo-dentin complex response to a resin-modified glass-ionomer cement and a bonding agent applied in deep cavities. Dent Mater. 2003;19(8):739–46.
20. de Souza Costa CA, Teixeira HM, Lopes do Nascimento AB, Hebling J. Biocompatibility of resin-based dental materials applied as liners in deep cavities prepared in human teeth. J Biomed Mater Res B Appl Biomater. 2007;81(1):175–84.
21. Modena KC, Casas-Apayco LC, Atta MT, Costa CAS, Hebling J, Sipert CR, Navarro MF, Santos CF. Cytotoxicity and biocompatibility of direct and indirect pulp capping materials. J Appl Oral Sci. 2009;17(6):544–54.
22. Costa CAS, Ribeiro AP, Giro EM, Randall RC, Hebling J. Pulp response after application of two resin modified glass ionomer cements (RMGICs) in deep cavities of prepared human teeth. Dent Mater. 2011;27(7):e158–70. doi:10.1016/j.dental.2011.04.002. Epub 2011 May 5.
23. About I, Murray PE, Franquin JC, Remusat M, Smith AJ. The effect of cavity restoration variables on odontoblast cell numbers and dental repair. J Dent. 2001;29:109–17.
24. Camps J, Dejou J, Remusat M, About I. Factors influencing pulpal response to cavity restorations. Dent Mater. 2000;16:432–40.
25. de Souza Costa CA, Hebling J, Randall RC. Human pulp response to resin cements used to bond inlay restorations. Dent Mater. 2006;22(10):954–62. Epub 2006 Jan 4.
26. Sloan AJ, Smith AJ. Stimulation of the dentine–pulp complex of rat incisor teeth by transforming growth factor-beta isoforms 1–3 *in vitro*. Arch Oral Biol. 1999;44:149–56.
27. Goldberg M, Smith AJ. Cells and extracellular matrices of dentin and pulp: a biological basis for repair and tissue engineering. Crit Rev Oral Biol Med. 2004;15:13–27.
28. Tecles O, Laurent P, Zygouritsas S, Burger AS, Camps J, Dejou J, About I. Activation of human dental pulp progenitor/stem cells in response to odontoblast injury. Arch Oral Biol. 2005;50:103–8.
29. Murray PE, About I, Lumley PJ, Franquin JC, Remusat M, Smith AJ. Cavity remaining dentin thickness and pulpal activity. Am J Dent. 2002;15:41–6.
30. Duque C, Negrini TC, Sacono NT, Spolidorio DM, de Souza Costa CA, Hebling J. Clinical and microbiological performance of resin-modified glass-ionomer liners after incomplete dentine caries removal. Clin Oral Investig. 2009;13(4):465–71. doi:10.1007/s00784-009-0304-2. Epub 2009 Jun 23.
31. Ruch JV, Lesot H, Begue-Kim C. Odontoblast differentiation. Inter J Develop Biol. 1995;39:51–68.

Clinical Pulpal Diagnosis

3

Marcio Guelmann

Contents

As of today, very little or no correlation exists between clinical diagnostic findings and the histopathologic status of the pulp [1]. Technologically advanced tests and tools to indicate the vitality condition of the pulp, such as laser Doppler flowmetry and pulse oximetry, are available. However, even these new technologies may lead to unreliable response when providing dental care for very young children and/or for patients with special health-care needs, due to uncooperative behavior.

Comprehensive medical history, thorough extra- and intraoral examinations, pain characteristics, and sensibility tests complemented by selected radiographs will provide the clinician with essential information regarding the pulp status of a particular tooth or teeth in question. In addition, the source of the discomfort, e.g., trauma or caries, and the presence of large, deep, or failed restorations also play a critical role in pulpal diagnosis and, subsequently, on the prognosis of the treatment to be provided.

M. Guelmann, DDS
Department of Pediatric Dentistry, University of Florida,
1395 Center Drive, Gainesville, FL 32610-0426, USA
e-mail: mguelmann@dental.ufl.edu

A.B. Fuks, B. Peretz (eds.), *Pediatric Endodontics: Current Concepts in Pulp Therapy for Primary and Young Permanent Teeth*,
DOI 10.1007/978-3-319-27553-6_3

In this chapter, all different elements contributing to the clinician in reaching an accurate pulp diagnosis will be discussed separately. At the end, the gathered information should be integrated to facilitate the clinical decision-making and the determination of the best treatment to be rendered.

3.1 Medical History

A child with a systemic disease needs a different approach than a healthy one [2]. Despite lack of evidence, for severely immunocompromised patients, the American Academy of Pediatric Dentistry (AAPD) recommends cautious considerations when treating deep carious lesions with close proximity to the pulp. When the pulp is involved, most clinicians decide to perform a more radical procedure such as an extraction, rather than performing a conservative treatment dealing with the risk of infections which might be life threatening. However, with existing pulpally treated teeth, periodic monitoring for signs of internal resorption or failure due to pulpal/periapical/furcal infections is recommended [3].

3.2 Extra- and Intraoral Examination

The presence of extraoral facial swelling, redness, and/or submandibular lymphadenopathy may indicate the presence of an acute dentoalveolar abscess (Fig. 3.1). In severe situations, facial cellulitis may involve the infraorbital space resulting in partial/total closure of the eye, limited mouth opening, fever, and malaise. Hospital admission for IV antibiotics may be necessary. Careful intraoral and radiographic examination seeking teeth with deep carious lesions or deep restorations must be performed (Fig. 3.2a–c). The diagnosis of pulp necrosis is then reached, and treatment decision of extraction or root canal therapy is based on the restorability of the tooth, severity of the infection, assessment of bone loss, lesion proximity to the succedaneous tooth follicle, and patient cooperation (Fig. 3.3). If the dental infection is contained within the pulpal tissue or the immediate surrounding tissue and the child patient presents no signs of systemic involvement such as fever or swelling, the use of antibiotic treatment is not indicated. This recommendation aims to minimize the risk of developing resistance to current antibiotic regimens [4].

During intraoral examination, the clinician should perform a careful soft tissue assessment searching for signs of swelling of the vestibule, presence of sinus tracts which may be associated with teeth affected by trauma (Fig. 3.4), caries, or deep restorations in close proximity to the pulp (Fig. 3.5a–d).

When examining hard tissues, teeth with questionable diagnosis should be evaluated for abnormal mobility and sensitivity to percussion. With the presence of open proximal carious lesions between adjacent teeth, the space can serve as reservoir

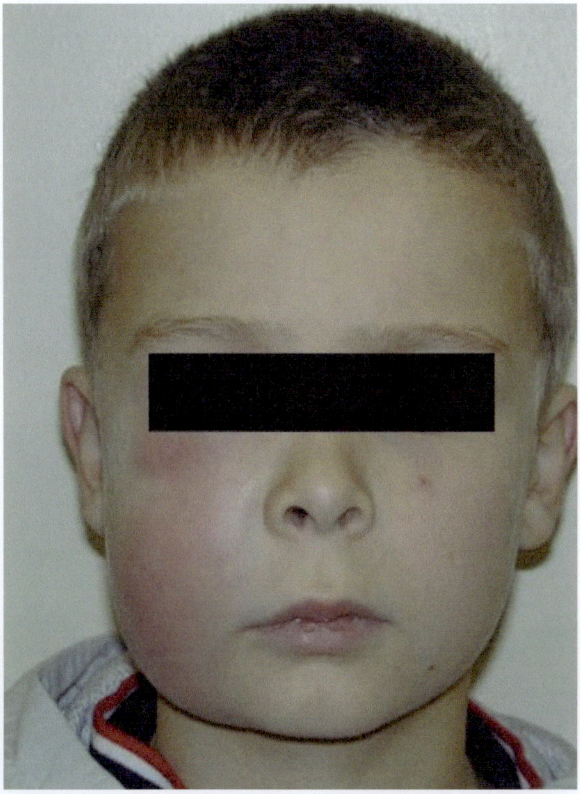

Fig. 3.1 Facial swelling and cellulitis as result of dentoalveolar abscess affecting maxillary primary molar (Courtesy of Dr. Abi Adewumi, University of Florida)

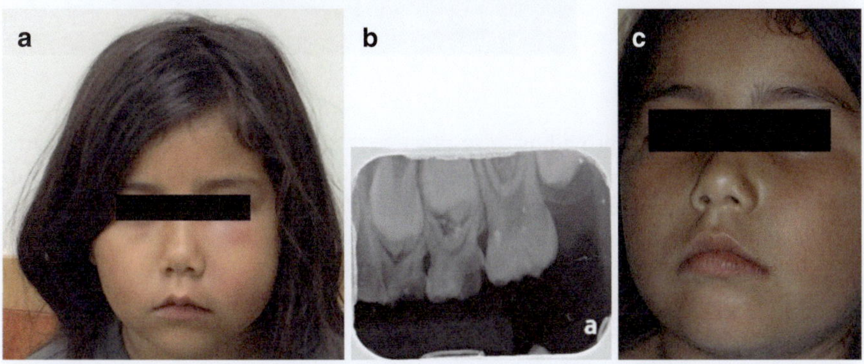

Fig. 3.2 (**a**) Facial cellulitis involving buccal and infraorbital space of a 7-year-old patient; (**b**) periapical radiograph reveals deep caries lesion affecting teeth #64 and #65 which are non-restorable; (**c**) normal facial appearance 6 days post-extraction of affected teeth (Courtesy of Dr. Chelsea Brinkman, Pediatric Dental Resident, University of Florida)

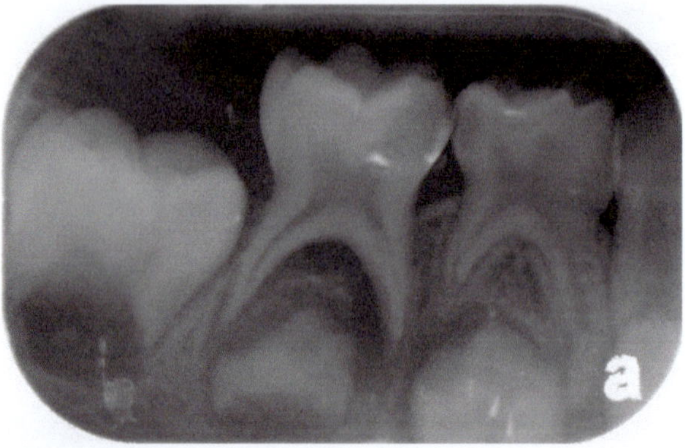

Fig. 3.3 Deep carious lesion of tooth #85 with large furcation and periapical involvement with close proximity to developing second premolar

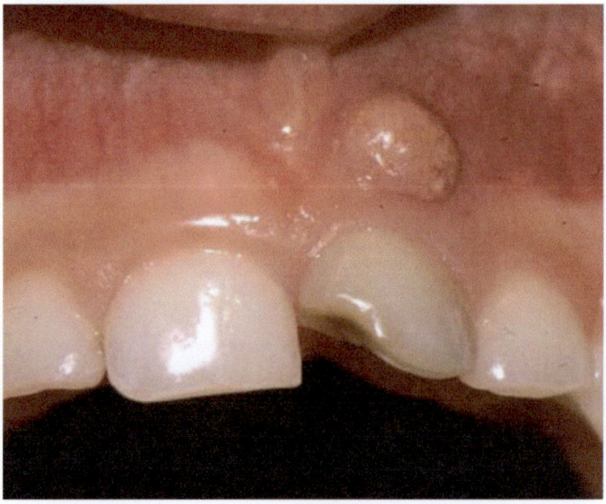

Fig. 3.4 Traumatic injury affecting tooth #61 resulting in discoloration, pulp necrosis, and sinus tract

causing food impaction providing false-positive response to percussion test (inflammation of interdental papilla rather than acute pulpal inflammation). In order to avoid behavior management problems, when performing percussion and palpation tests in children, the tip of the finger should be gently used in combination with Tell, Show, and Do (TSD) technique [5]. The clinician should start the test with a contralateral non-affected tooth to familiarize the patient with a normal response to the stimuli.

3.3 Pain Characteristics

Young children are not good historians. For this group, parents are the ones better prepared to reporting existing symptoms. Stimuli-related responses that cease when the insult is removed (provoked or elicited pain) generally indicate a favorable,

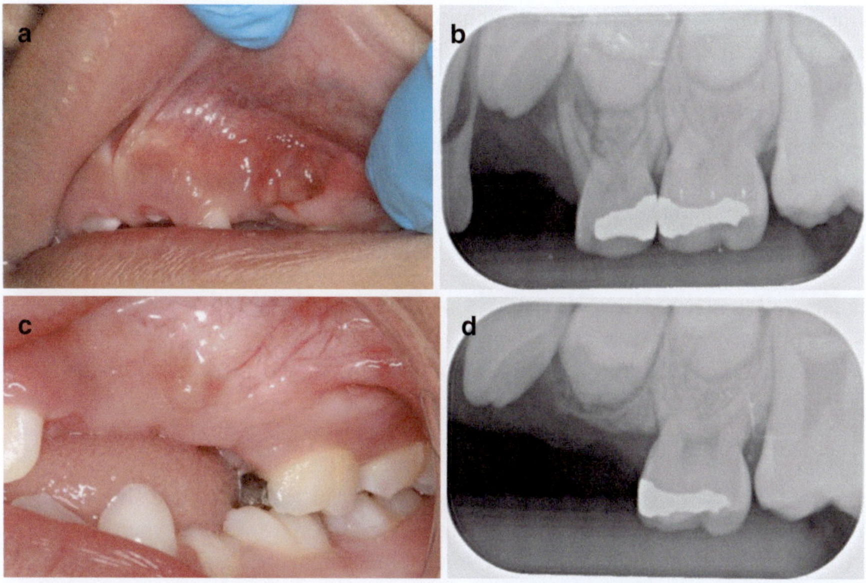

Fig. 3.5 (**a**, **b**) Intraoral sinus tract caused by a necrotic pulp and a deep amalgam restoration on tooth #54. Note that the crown is partially covered by the lower lip. (**c**, **d**) Healing of the area after extraction of tooth # 54, 10 weeks' post-extraction (Courtesy of Dr. Jeffery Jackson, Pediatric Dental Resident, University of Florida)

reversible status of the pulp which could lead to a more conservative treatment approach such as indirect pulp therapy (IPT) or pulpotomy. Complaints of persistent, lingering, or throbbing pain disturbing sleep and preventing regular activity are generally referred as "spontaneous pain." This most probably indicates an irreversible status of the pulp. The information in combination with clinical examination and radiographic image(s) will lead the clinician to treatment options such as pulpectomy or extraction.

3.4 Sensibility Tests

Sensibility and percussion tests are not indicated in primary teeth due to inconsistent results [6]. Younger patients may also be more anxious and less reliable because of the subjective nature of the test [7]. The most commonly used pulpal sensibility tests are cold and electric pulp tester (EPT) [7, 8]. For a reliable response, teeth need to be dried and well isolated. Adjacent and/or contralateral teeth to the one in question are generally tested first, as controls, to observe a baseline normal response. Refrigerant spray is the most commonly used. It is convenient, user-friendly, and reliable with a level of accuracy higher than EPT [7, 9, 10]. The cold test may be used to differentiate between reversible and irreversible pulpitis. If pain subsides when the stimulus is removed, a diagnosis of reversible pulpitis is appropriate. If a lingering pain persists, irreversible pulpitis is more likely [11]. Jespersen et al. evaluated the pulpal response to cold and EPT in the presence and absence of caries. They found that presence of caries in vital teeth resulted in a more accurate response to cold testing. However, *no response* to cold on carious teeth makes a diagnosis of pulpal necrosis more accurate [7]. Patients in early mixed dentition and with deep carious lesions affecting permanent molars well tolerated cold test as proof of pulpal vitality before caries excavation [12].

3.5 Preoperative Diagnosis of Deep Caries Lesions

When facing deep carious lesions affecting the primary dentition, limitations exist regarding the determination of the vitality status of the pulp. Percussion and palpations tests, combined with bitewing and selected periapical radiographs, are complimentary information that must be obtained. Good quality bitewing radiographs showing clearly the furcation area are essential for an accurate diagnosis. However, in young children in primary and early mixed dentition, especially when using size #0 or #1 films, visibility of the apical third of the primary molar roots and the apical formation of first permanent molars is not always possible. In these situations, a periapical radiograph should be obtained to rule out the presence of internal resorption or periapical involvement. Figure 3.6a shows a left bitewing of an asymptomatic tooth #75 with a deep carious lesion. The supplemental periapical radiograph discloses neither furcation nor periapical pathology, indicating good prognosis for a conservative pulp treatment such as IPT (Fig. 3.6b). Conversely, a periapical radiograph reveals furcation pathology in tooth # 85, indicating pulp necrosis, not evident in a bitewing (Fig. 3.6c, d). In Fig. 3.6e, internal root resorption and furcation involvement can be observed in a periapical radiograph of a symptomatic tooth #85.

Success of pulpotomies performed previously in the primary molars of a 7-year-old patient can be observed in a bitewing radiograph. However, the visibility of the roots of the first permanent molar (#36) with a deep carious lesion is limited (Fig. 3.6f). A supplemental periapical radiograph reveals normal root development and absence of pathology (Fig. 3.6g).

Integrity and continuity of the lamina dura together with the presence of trabecular bone in the bifurcation area of primary molars are indicative signs of a vital pulp (Fig. 3.7).

Due to anatomical differences and superposition of images, clear visualizations of these structures may be difficult to obtain in the maxillary arch [2]. In asymptomatic primary and permanent teeth, the amount of sound dentin (at least 1.0 mm) separating the deepest layer of the caries lesion and the pulp horn can also play an important role when determining if a conservative approach such as IPT is recommended [13]. Recently, a clinical attempt to possibly assess pulpal diagnosis status of deep caries lesions affecting primary molars using interim therapeutic restorations has been advocated [14]. This technique will be discussed in detail in Chap. 4.

For asymptomatic or teeth with reversible pulpal inflammation, in order to preserve dental structures and avoid further damage to the pulp, conservative approaches

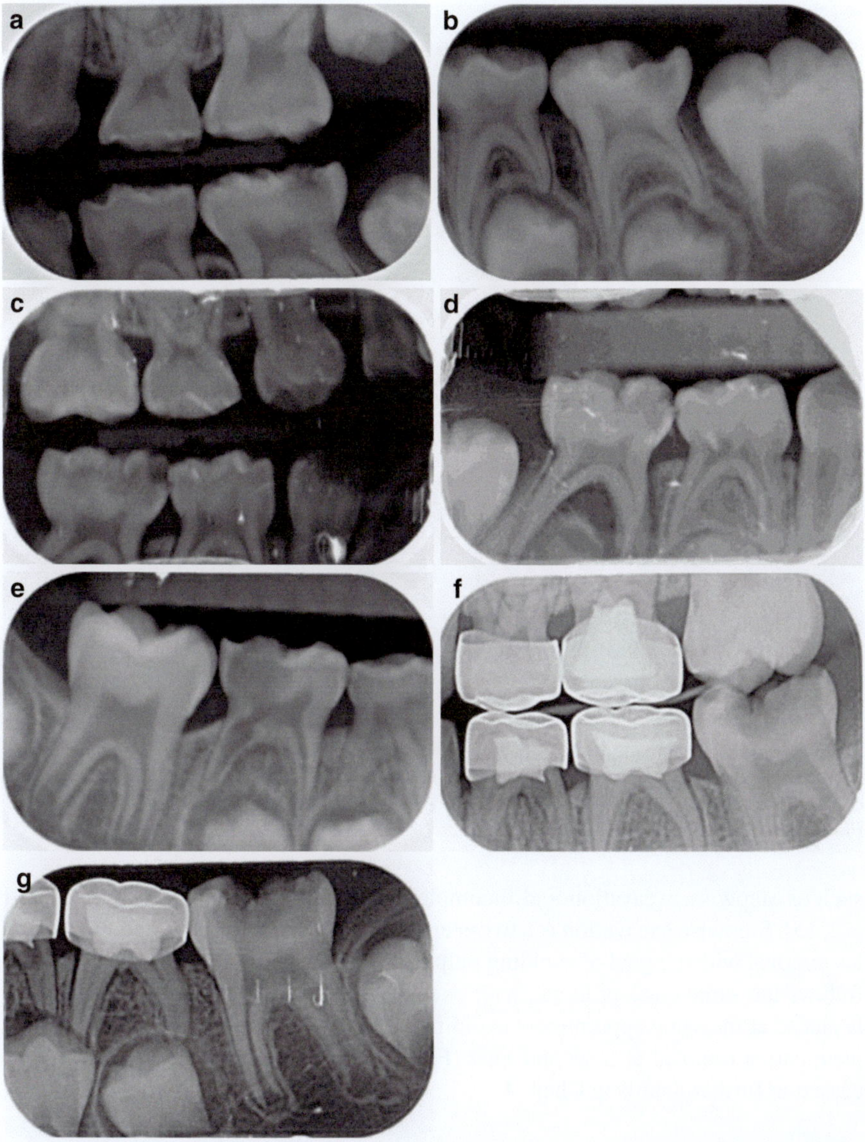

Fig. 3.6 (**a**) Left bitewing of an asymptomatic tooth #75 with a deep carious lesion; (**b**) periapical radiograph reveals no furcation pathology indicating good prognosis for a conservative pulp treatment such as IPT. (**c**) Right bitewing of a 4-year-old patient with spontaneous pain affecting tooth #85 which is sensitive to percussion; (**d**) a periapical radiograph reveals furcation pathology indicating pulp necrosis; (**e**) on a different patient, but a similar situation, a periapical radiograph of symptomatic tooth #85 showing internal root resorption and furcation involvement. (**f**) Bitewing radiograph of a 7-year-old patient showing limited visibility of the roots of the first permanent molar (#36) with a deep carious lesion. (**g**) A supplemental periapical radiograph reveals normal root development and absence of pathology (Courtesy of Dr. Nicole Eastham, Pediatric Dental Resident, University of Florida)

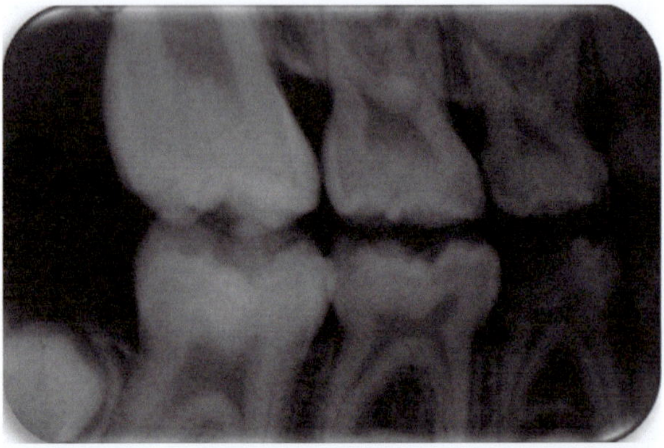

Fig. 3.7 Deep carious lesion affecting tooth #84. Tooth is asymptomatic, lamina dura is continuous, and furcation area is filled with trabecular bone

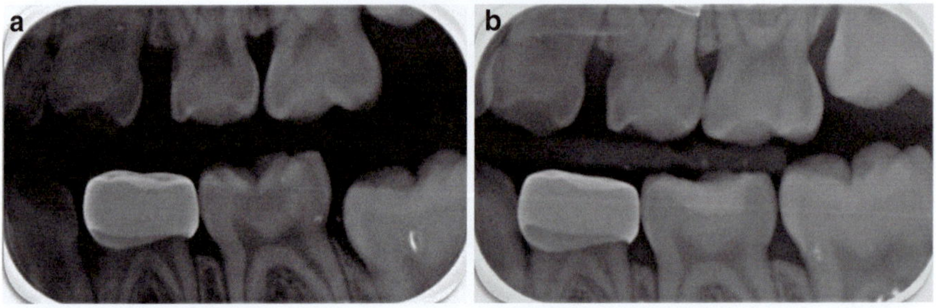

Fig. 3.8 (**a**) Asymptomatic tooth #75 with deep carious lesion treated with incomplete caries excavation and a composite resin restoration; (**b**) 6 months later, healing of the pulp by formation of reparative dentin (Courtesy of Dr. Susana Perry, Pediatric Dental Resident, University of Florida)

such as stepwise excavation and incomplete caries removal should be considered [12, 15]. Stepwise excavation is a two-step, conservative approach for complete caries removal with the goal of avoiding pulp exposure [15]. Incomplete caries removal follows the same concept as stepwise excavation; however, a definitive restoration is placed at the same appointment avoiding the risk of a pulp exposure during complete caries removal at a second visit (Fig. 3.8a, b). Both techniques will be discussed in further details in Chap. 4.

3.6 Operative Diagnosis

There are instances when a final diagnosis can only be achieved by direct evaluation of the pulp tissue and a decision about treatment is made accordingly. The quality (color) and the amount of bleeding from a direct exposure of the pulp tissue must be assessed; profuse bleeding or purulent exudate indicates irreversible pulpitis or pulpal necrosis. Based on these observations, the treatment plan may be confirmed or changed. For example, if a formocresol pulpotomy is

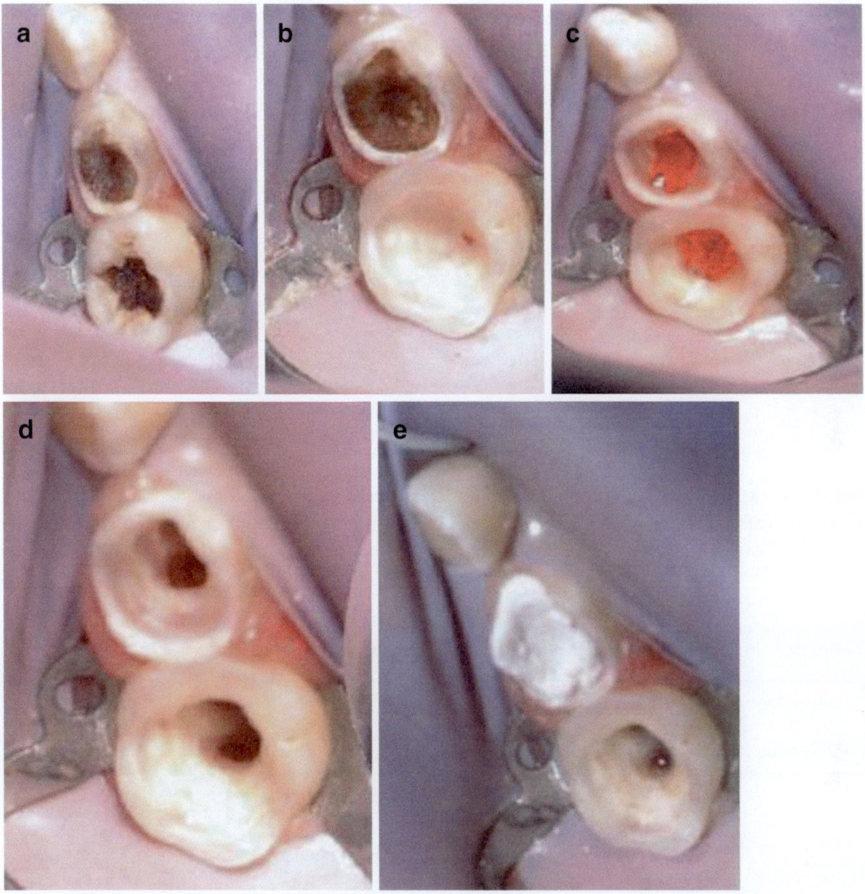

Fig. 3.9 (**a**) First and second primary molars with extensive caries. (**b**) Pulp exposure after complete caries removal. (**c**) Extensive bleeding after pulp amputation; the color of the blood is *bright red*. (**d**) Bleeding stopped, indicating the tooth is appropriate for a pulpotomy. (**e**) The pulp stumps are covered with a ZOE paste (Courtesy of Nathan Rozenfarb, DMD)

planned, the nature of the bleeding from the amputation site should be normal (red color and hemostasis evident in less than 5 min with mild cotton pellet pressure). If bleeding persists, a more radical treatment should be undertaken (pulpectomy or extraction). Excessive bleeding is an indication that the inflammation has reached the radicular pulp. Conversely, if a pulp polyp is present and bleeding stops normally after coronal pulp amputation, a pulpotomy may be performed instead of a more radical procedure (Fig. 3.9a–e) [16]. Direct pulp capping of carious pulp-exposed primary teeth is not recommended due to questionable prognosis [3].

For young immature permanent teeth with vital pulp, direct pulp capping, partial pulpotomy, and cervical pulpotomy are indicated treatments (Fig. 3.10a–c).

If the diagnosis of pulp necrosis is made, apexification and pulp regeneration techniques are recommended approaches to induce closure of the apex. In depth, discussion of these techniques will take place in Chap. 8.

A schematic diagram for pulpal diagnosis in primary and young permanent teeth affected by deep carious lesions is presented in Tables 3.1 and 3.2.

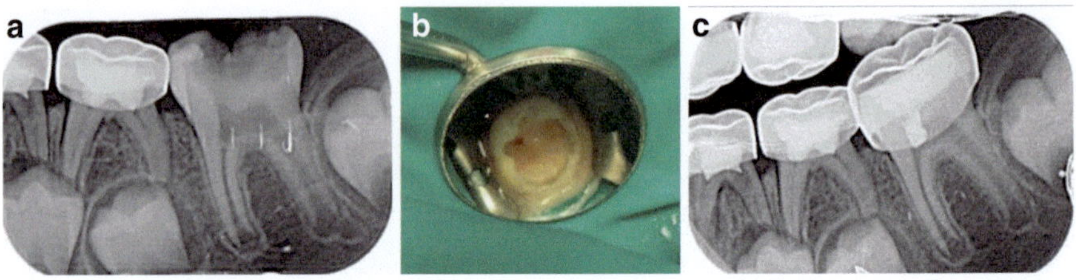

Fig. 3.10 (**a**) Tooth #36 with reversible pulpitis; (**b**) caries excavation resulted in pinpoint pulp exposure; (**c**) tooth #36, asymptomatic, 3 months after partial pulpotomy with MTA (Courtesy of Dr. Nicole Eastham, Pediatric Dental Resident, University of Florida)

Table 3.1 Pulpal diagnosis tree for deep carious lesions in primary teeth

Pain History:	Asymptomatic/Elicited/Provoked	Spontaneous
Pulp Status:	(Possibly Reversible)	(Possibly Irreversible)

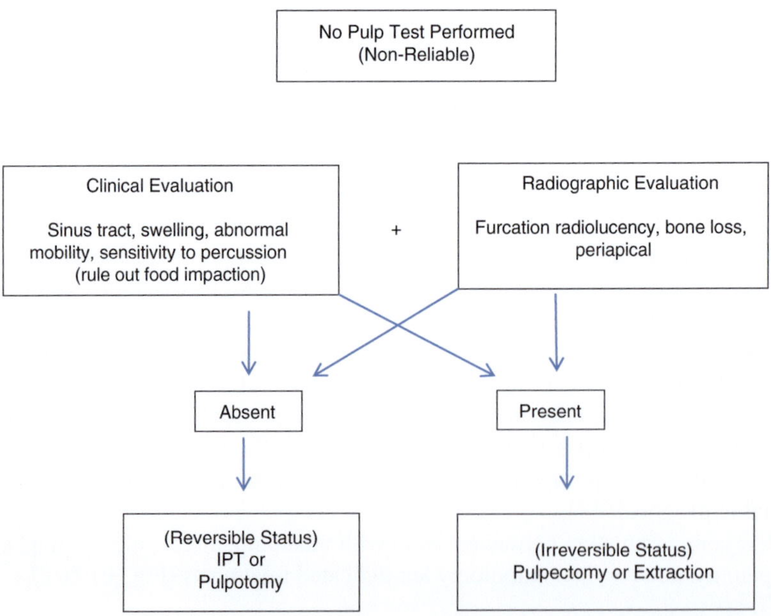

Table 3.2 Pulpal diagnosis tree for deep carious lesions in immature permanent teeth

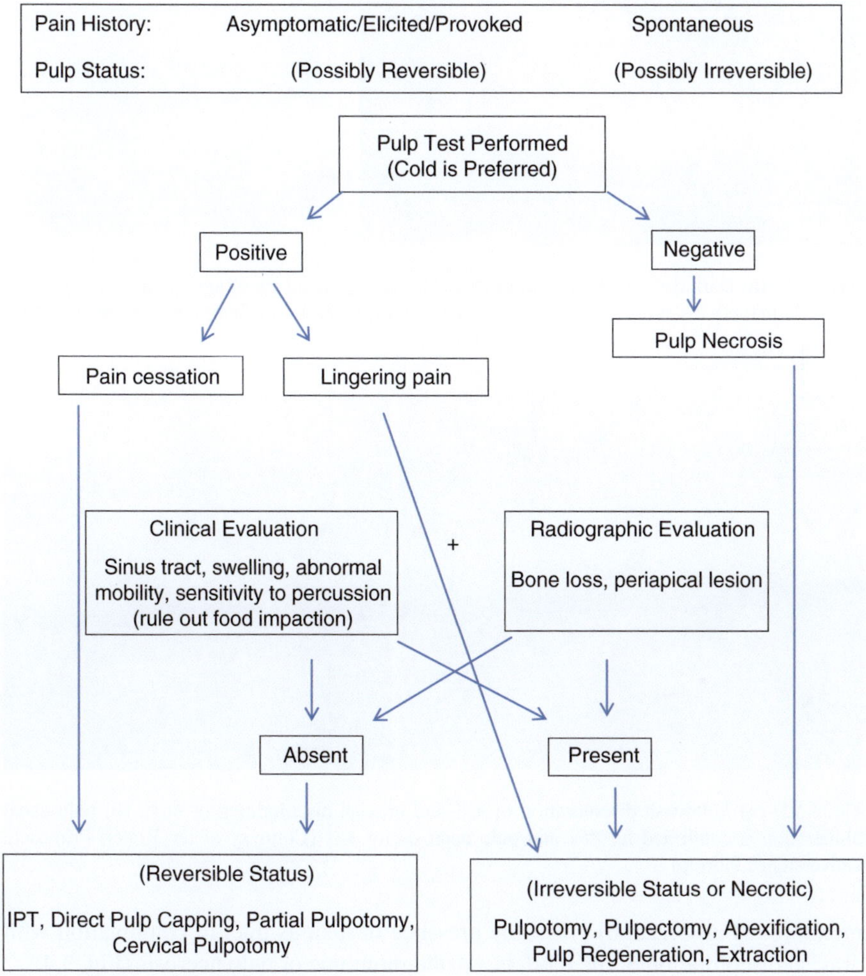

3.7 Trauma

Traumatic injuries to primary and young permanent dentitions can have an impact on the vitality status of the pulp. Discoloration of the crown may indicate internal changes in the pulp canal. Yellow and grayish colors are the most commonly found as sequelae of traumatic injuries. Periapical radiographs will aid on the diagnosis and determination of treatment if needed. Teeth diagnosed with pulp canal obliteration (yellowish) are vital and should be periodically monitored (Fig. 3.11a–b).

Teeth with light/dark gray discoloration may or may not be necrotic. If asymptomatic and no signs of soft tissue and/or periapical pathology, they should be only,

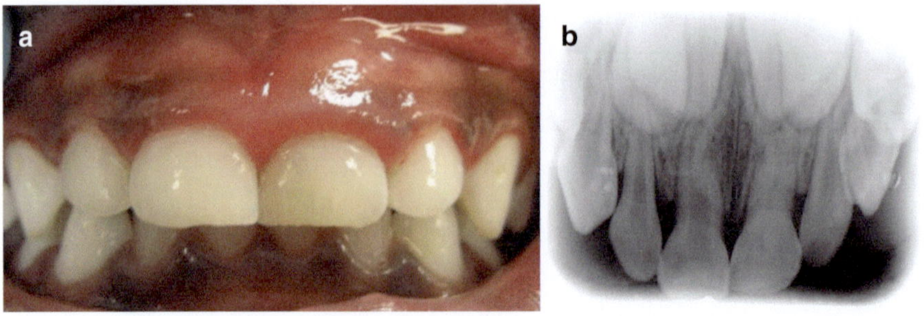

Fig. 3.11 (**a**) Dark discoloration of tooth #61. Mother was unaware of any trauma and was concerned with tooth discoloration; (**b**) revealed pulp canal obliteration affecting #61. Tooth is asymptomatic, normal PDL, and continuous lamina dura

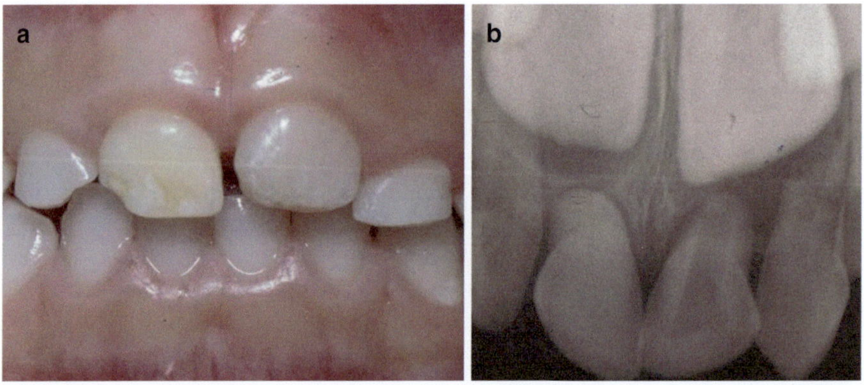

Fig. 3.12 (**a**) Yellowish discoloration of #51 and grayish discoloration of #61;, (**b**) pulp canal obliteration is confirmed for #51 and pulp necrosis for #61 (Courtesy of Dr. Robert Primosch, University of Florida)

monitored (Fig. 3.12a, b) [17]. The presence of a sinus tract in combination with grayish discoloration of the tooth is a pathognomonic of pulp necrosis (Fig. 3.4).

After traumatic injuries affecting permanent teeth, the accuracy of sensibility tests is low. A temporary loss of response is expected especially with luxation-like injuries. EPT provides the best support for pulpal diagnosis after long-term follow-up [10].

Sensibility tests have their limitations. These tests check for sensory response to the injury, but do not assess vascularity of the pulp [18]. Pulse oximetry and laser Doppler flowmetry are examples of tests that, respectively, analyze the oxygen saturation and blood flow to the tooth. Their applicability is important when temporary paresthesia of nerves occurs, reducing the reliability of thermal and electric pulp tests [8]. However, due to high cost of the laser Doppler flowmetry device [2] and the need to develop a commercially tooth-adaptable probe (pulse oximeter), these tests are not routinely used today. With rapid advances in knowledge and technology, more accurate and predictable means of assessing pulp vitality will be available [11].

The stage of root formation has an important role in the diagnosis and prognosis of the pulp. Due to their high vascularity, immature teeth have better healing potential than when their apices are closed. This subject will be dealt in more detail in Chap. 8.

3.8 Correlation Between Histopathologic Status of the Pulp and Deep Caries

In primary teeth, very few studies investigated the correlation between caries depth and the degree of pulpal inflammation. Eidelman and Ulmansky [19] assessed the histologic appearance of the pulp of decayed, extracted, non-restorable primary incisors affected by early childhood caries. Caries removal was performed resulting or not in pulp exposures. When pulp exposure did not occur, pulps were more likely to be normal. It was concluded that absence of pulp exposure could be a good indicator of a normal histologic status of the pulp. In cases when the pulp was exposed, most teeth had inflammation confined to the coronal pulp and were considered good candidates for pulpotomy. Kassa et al. [20] investigated the pulp inflammation status of extracted primary molars with occlusal and proximal caries. They found that when decay extended more than 50 % of dentin thickness, more extensive pulpal inflammation was noted for proximal caries lesions than for occlusal ones with similar depth. A recent study using well-defined criteria for clinic and histologic classifications of pulp conditions on extracted permanent teeth revealed a good agreement when the diagnosis of normal and reversible pulpitis was made prior to tooth extraction [21].

3.9 Summary

Only integration of the gathered clinical and radiographic information will give the clinician a direction to achieve the most accurate diagnosis possible. Clinical pulpal diagnosis continues to be a field where more investigation is needed to develop conclusive tests to help the clinician with accurate decision-making. This statement is supported by a recent systematic review of the literature revealing overall insufficient evidence to obtain an accurate diagnosis of the condition of the pulp [22].

Important Things to Remember

- Young patients are not good historians. Parents should be inquired during pain history data collection.
- Sensibility tests are not performed in primary teeth.
- For young patients, percussion and palpation tests should be performed gently to prevent disruptive behavior.
- Cold test with refrigerant spray should be used in immature permanent teeth affected by deep caries lesions to determine the reversible status of the pulp.
- Good quality bitewing and periapical radiographs are essential for the disclosure of pathology affecting the furcation and/or the periapical area.

References

1. Levin LC, Law AS, Holland GR, Abbott PV, Roda RS. Identify and define all diagnostic terms for pulpal health and disease status. J Endod. 2009;35:1645–57.
2. Camp JH. Diagnosis dilemmas in vital pulp therapy: treatment for the toothache is changing, especially in young, immature teeth. Pediatr Dent. 2008;30:197–205.
3. American Academy of Pediatric Dentistry Reference Manual. Guideline on pulp therapy for primary and immature permanent teeth. Pediatr Dent. 2014–2015;36:242–50.
4. American Academy of Pediatric Dentistry Reference Manual. Guideline on use of antibiotic therapy for pediatric dental patients. Pediatr Dent. 2014–2015;36:284–6.
5. Fuks AB. Pulp therapy for the primary dentition. In: Pinkham JR, editor. Pediatric dentistry: infancy through adolescence. Philadelphia: Saunders; 2005.
6. Malmgren B, Andreasen JO, Flores MT, Robertson A, DiAngelis AJ, Andersson L, Cavalleri G, Cohenca N, Day P, Hicks LM, Malmgren O, Moule AJ, Onetto J, Tsukiboshi M. Guidelines for the management traumatic dental injuries: 3. Injuries in the primary dentition. Dent Traumatol. 2012;28:174–82.
7. Jespersen JJ, Hellstein J, Williamson A, Johnson WT, Qian F. Evaluation of dental pulp sensibility tests in a clinical setting. J Endod. 2014;40:351–4.
8. Gopikrishna V, Tinagupta K, Kandaswamy D. Comparison of electrical, thermal, and pulse oximetry methods for assessing pulp vitality in recently traumatized teeth. J Endod. 2007;33:531–5.
9. Villa-Chavez CE, Patiño-Marín N, Loyola-Rodriguez JP, Zavala-Alonso NV, Martínez-Castañón GA, Medina-Solís CE. Predictive values of thermal and electric dental pulp tests: a clinical study. J Endod. 2013;39:965–069.
10. Bastos JV, Goulart MAG, Cortes MLS. Pulpal response to sensibility tests after traumatic dental injuries in permanent teeth. Dent Traumatol. 2014;30:188–92.
11. Gopikrishna V, Pradeep G, Venkatesh babu N. Assessment of pulp vitality: a review. Int J Paediatr Dent. 2009;19:3–15.
12. Maltz M, Jardim JJ, Mestrinho HD, Yamaguti PM, Podestá K, Moura MS, de Paula LM. Partial removal of carious dentine: a multicenter randomized controlled trial and 18-month follow-up results. Caries Res. 2013;47:103–9.
13. Reeves R, Stainley HR. The relationship of bacteria penetration and pulpal pathosis in carious teeth. Oral Surg Oral Med Oral Pathol. 1966;22:59–65.
14. Coll JA, Campbell A, Chalmers NI. Effects of glass ionomer temporary restorations on pulpal diagnosis and treatment outcomes in primary molars. Pediatr Dent. 2013;35:416–21.
15. Bjørndal L. Indirect pulp therapy and stepwise excavation. Pediatr Dent. 2010;30:225–9.
16. Fuks A, Guelmann M, Kupietzky A. Currents developments in pulp therapy for primary teeth. Endod Top. 2012;23:50–72.
17. Holan G. Long-term effect of different treatment modalities for traumatized primary incisors presenting dark coronal discoloration with no other signs of injury. Dent Traumatol. 2006;22:14–7.
18. Jafarzade H, Rosenberg PA. Pulse oximetry: review of a potential aid in endodontic diagnosis. J Endod. 2009;35:329–33.
19. Eidelman E, Ulmansky M. Histopathology of the pulp in primary incisors with deep dentinal caries. Pediatr Dent. 1992;14:372–5.
20. Kassa A, Day P, High A, Duggal M. Histological comparison of pulpal inflammation in primary teeth with occlusal or proximal caries. Int J Paediatr Dent. 2009;19:26–33.
21. Ricucci A, Loghin S, Siqueira JF. Correlation between clinical and histologic pulp diagnoses. J Endod. 2014;40:1932–9.
22. Mejàre IA, Axelsson S, Davidson T, Frisk F, Hakeberg M, Kvist T, Norlund A, Petersson A, Portenier I, Sandberg H, Tranaeus S, Bergenholtz G. Diagnosis of the condition of the pulp: a systematic review. Int Endod J. 2012;45:597–613.

Indirect Pulp Treatment, Direct Pulp Capping, and Stepwise Caries Excavation

4

James A. Coll

Contents

J.A. Coll, DMD, MS
Division of Pediatric Dentistry, University of Maryland School of Dentistry,
Baltimore, MD, USA
e-mail: dmd1@comcast.net

A.B. Fuks, B. Peretz (eds.), *Pediatric Endodontics: Current Concepts in Pulp Therapy for Primary and Young Permanent Teeth*,
DOI 10.1007/978-3-319-27553-6_4

4.1 Purpose of Chapter

4.1.1 Goal: To Use IPT Vital Pulp Treatment to Preserve Pulp Vitality

Many practitioners believe that for primary teeth, when the carious lesion is within 1 mm or less of the pulp, a pulpotomy must be the treatment of choice, if the pulp is judged to be vital. Chap. 5 will discuss pulpotomy and its advantages and disadvantages. The alternative treatment for this scenario is indirect pulp treatment (*IPT*), also termed indirect pulp capping, when the pulp is vital [1]. This chapter will describe a reliable method to diagnose the primary tooth's pulp vitality under deep caries prior to performing any vital pulp treatment [2]. In permanent teeth with deep carious lesions, direct pulp capping is an alternative if a pinpoint pulp exposure is caused doing complete caries excavation in an asymptomatic tooth [1] (see Chaps. 3 and 8). The indications for direct pulp capping for primary and permanent teeth will be presented, and the relevant literature will be reviewed. For an immature permanent tooth, preserving pulp vitality is critically important to allow complete root formation and thickening of the pulpal walls [3]. IPT is highly indicated for treating deep carious lesions in immature and mature permanent teeth, and studies have shown its reliable success rate. Focusing on complete, stepwise, and partial caries excavation, this chapter will address the importance of the choice of caries excavation for IPT success. Many studies have examined the base or medicament used for IPT. This chapter will review the studies in this area to give a clear choice as to the liner of choice.

4.2 Definitions (See Chap. 2 for Details)

Tertiary dentin is the dentin formed as a reaction to an external stimulus like dental caries. It can be of two types: reactionary or reparative dentin [4].

Reactionary dentin is formed from the original odontoblasts as a reaction to a stimulus like caries [4].

Reparative dentin is formed when the caries is deep and close to the pulp, so the odontoblasts are killed off and odontoblastic-like cells form dentin that is atubular [4].

Infected dentin is the outer layer of carious dentin, which is infected with bacteria [5].

Affected dentin is the inner layer of carious dentin which is demineralized but largely uninfected with bacteria [6].

Indirect pulp treatment also termed *indirect pulp capping* is the vital pulp treatment where the deepest decay is left in place to avoid a pulp exposure and the tooth restored to prevent microleakage [1].

4.3 The Dental Caries Process

Dental caries is initiated as a white spot lesion on the enamel surface. The pulp responds by altering the dentin in the area under the white spot. Bjorndal [7] described the pulp reaction in the odontoblasts: He stated that the size of the odontoblasts decreases

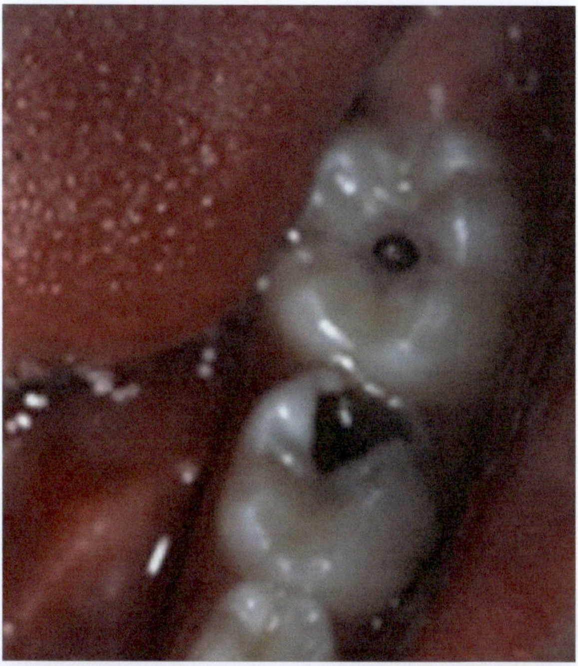

Fig. 4.1 An open lesion in the distal of the second primary molar is slower growing and dark in color. The first permanent molar has a closed lesion which progresses faster, is moist, and has a yellowish color inside (Photograph courtesy of Dr. N Sue Seale)

initially compared to odontoblasts unaffected by decay. As the enamel demineralization deepens, the dentin under that area becomes hypermineralized and sclerotic under the localized area of enamel demineralization [8]. Dentin demineralization begins only when enamel decalcification contacts the dentin-enamel junction [9]. Cavitation of the tooth surface occurs when the demineralized enamel crumbles, allowing bacteria to begin their invasion into the enamel [7]. The dentin in an active lesion is yellow, and its hardness is lower compared to normal dentin. Arrested lesions have dark and harder dentin. Bjorndal also defined an open and closed carious lesion [7] (Fig. 4.1).

The closed lesion has a homogeneous mixture of lactobacillus subspecies and progresses faster while the open lesion has many different bacterial species and is slower growing [10]. The clinical implication from cariology for a closed lesion is that caries progress is accelerated and may not allow reparative dentin formation to prevent the caries reaching the pulp quickly. Proper caries excavation, without removing the entire lesion, can avoid a pulp exposure. An open lesion progresses slower, usually allowing reparative dentin formation that can prevent pulp exposures [7].

4.4 Methods of Caries Excavation

4.4.1 Complete Excavation

Traditional operative dentistry approach to deep caries treatment advocated its total removal using slow-speed rotary burs and hand instruments [11]. Complete excavation removes all the infected and affected dentin.

4.4.1.1 Complete Excavation and Rate of Pulp Exposure

A pulp exposure can occur when complete excavation of deep caries is employed. A meta-analysis revealed that complete caries excavation of deep caries in primary and permanent teeth has three times the odds ratio of creating a pulp exposure compared to partial excavation [12]. Another systematic review of pulp exposures after complete excavation demonstrated that partial caries removal reduced the incidence of an exposure by 77 % compared to complete excavation [13].

In 1990, Elderton [14] claimed that most restorations were replacement restorations due to caries and/or restoration failure. This replacement of restorations could result in a very thin amount of dentin covering the pulp. The amount of remaining dentin under a restoration has been shown to be the most critical factor in determining the future health of the pulp [15] (see Chap. 2). In a closed carious lesion with extensive moist dentin, complete excavation will greatly thin out the remaining dentin. Therefore, over-excavation is not recommended [7].

4.4.1.2 Complete Excavation and Direct Pulp Capping for Primary Teeth

Performing direct pulp capping after complete excavation of deep caries is contraindicated in primary teeth due to the unreliable outcomes [16]. In addition, as described in Chap. 5, pulpotomy would likely be indicated and have a higher success rate. For a traumatic exposure or a mechanical exposure occurring during cavity preparation of shallow decay, performing a direct pulp capping with calcium hydroxide or mineral trioxide aggregate (MTA) is indicated [1].

4.4.1.3 Complete Excavation and Direct Pulp Capping for Permanent Teeth

Direct pulp capping after pulp exposures resulting from excavating deep caries has been shown to have low success in permanent teeth [17, 18]. In a randomized multicenter study on direct pulp capping or partial pulpotomy with calcium hydroxide involving 58 patients with exposed pulps after caries excavation in permanent teeth, the authors reported a low success rate (31.8 % vs. 34.5 %, respectively) and no significant difference in pulp vitality between the two pulp capping procedures after a 1-year or more follow-up [17]. Al-Hiyasat et al. [18] found that carious exposures had a 33 % pulp capping success compared to 92.2 % success for a mechanical exposure.

Another method for treating a pulp exposure after complete excavation in permanent teeth was described by Bogen et al. and had a much higher success [19]. In this retrospective report, the author recommended creating, on purpose, a large pulp exposure, rinsing extensively with sodium hypochlorite to control the bleeding, placing MTA on the pulp followed by a temporary filling. A second visit was required to place a final restoration. This procedure resulted in a 98 % success in 49 teeth after almost 4 years.

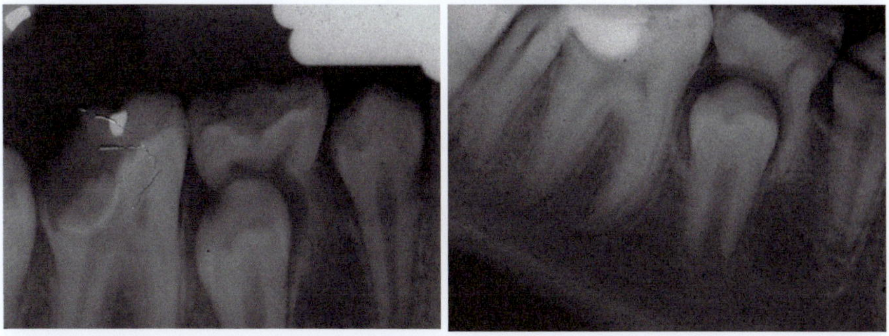

Fig. 4.2 Mandibular right first permanent molar presented with a history of pain when chewing foods of short duration (initial radiograph). No other signs or symptoms in this 12-year-old patient (*left*). Periapical film shows posttreatment first visit stepwise excavation with a calcium hydroxide base and a reinforced zinc oxide temporary filling in place (*right*)

4.4.2 Stepwise Caries Excavation (SW)

The second method of deep caries excavation is termed stepwise excavation and is done over two patient visits. The first excavation is intended to remove the superficial necrotic, infected, and affected dentin by completely excavating the periphery of the lesion. This excavation does not excavate caries near the pulp to avoid a pulp exposure [20]. A retentive temporary restoration is placed leaving soft, moist, discolored dentin on the pulpal floor. The dentin is then covered with calcium hydroxide and a self-setting glass ionomer temporary filling [17] (Fig. 4.2). A resin-modified glass ionomer has also been advocated in place of the self-setting glass ionomer [21]. SW is intended to allow remineralization of the affected dentin and formation of more tertiary dentin [20]. The carious lesion is reentered in 8–12 weeks by removing the temporary, and a final complete excavation is done leaving only central yellowish or grayish hard dentin in the pulpal floor (Fig. 4.3). A final restoration is placed with the intention to seal the pulp from any microleakage [17]. In two systematic reviews and meta-analysis studies [12, 13], SW significantly reduced pulp exposures compared to complete excavation (Fig. 4.4).

4.4.3 Partial (Incomplete) Caries Excavation

The third type of caries excavation is termed partial or incomplete excavation involving one appointment removal of the peripheral decay but intentionally leaving the deepest caries in place to avoid a pulp exposure. An indirect pulp treatment is then completed (Fig. 4.5).

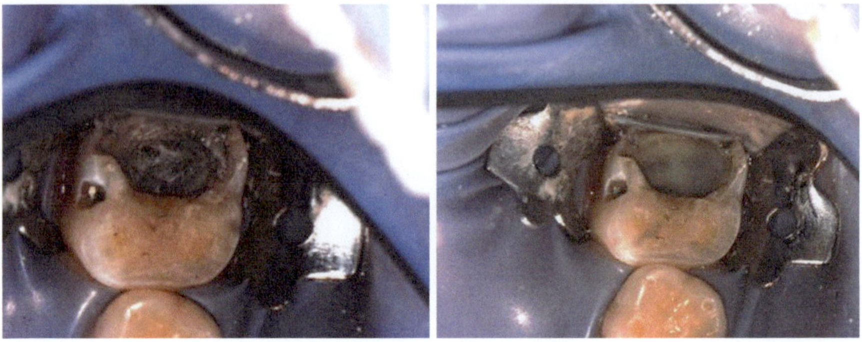

Fig. 4.3 Same mandibular first molar 8 weeks after the second stepwise excavation showing the hard dark dentin on the pulpal floor and the complete peripheral excavation (*left*). The right photograph shows a resin-modified glass ionomer base prior to steel crown placement

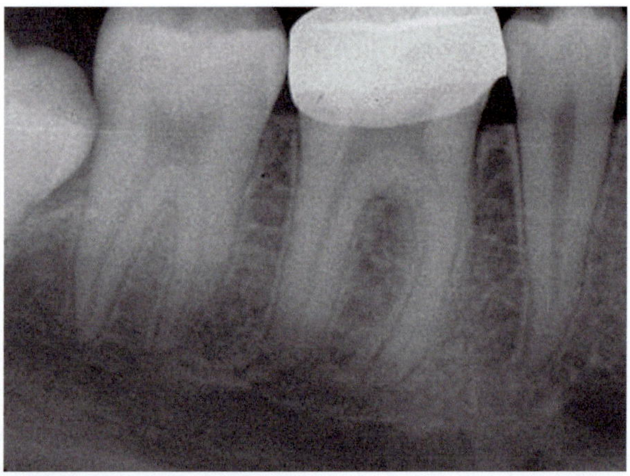

Fig. 4.4 Same mandibular permanent molar 48 months after stepwise excavation and indirect pulp treatment. The tooth was asymptomatic and the radiograph showed no pathology

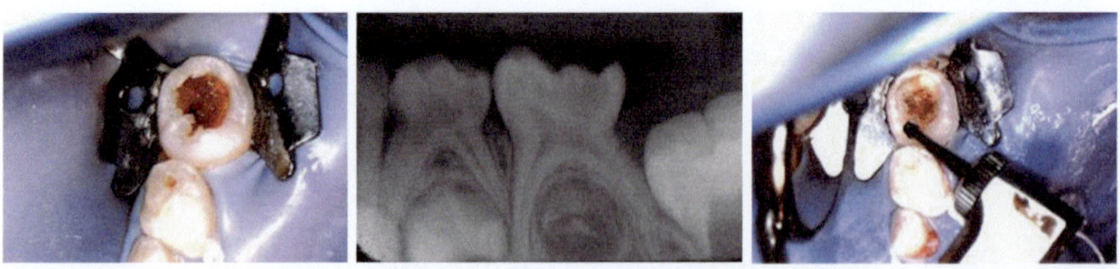

Fig. 4.5 Preoperative view (*left*) and radiograph (*center*) of a mandibular left second primary molar with deep dentinal caries. View of the partial excavation showing peripheral caries removed but the deeper caries is left in place (*right*). An indirect pulp treatment was then performed

Partial excavation omits the reentry and second excavation done in SW by sealing off the caries with a final restoration placed at the same appointment [12] (Fig. 4.6).

Partial excavation attempts to shift the microbial balance within the affected dentin to promote dentin remineralization and arrest the carious lesion [22].

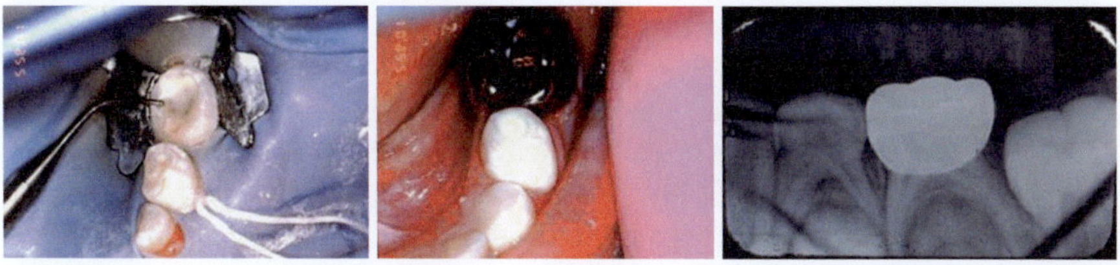

Fig. 4.6 Same second primary molar as Fig. 4.5 treated in one appointment showing a resin-modified glass ionomer base used as the IPT medicament (*left*) and then cementation of the steel crown with glass ionomer cement (*center*). The radiograph (*right*) shows the tooth 18 months later without history of pain, normal soft tissue, and no pathology

Maltz et al. [23, 24] published the results of one randomized controlled trial (RCT) comparing stepwise to partial excavation in 299 permanent molars in two time frames. The results of the 2- and 3-year follow-up showed significantly higher success rates of one appointment partial caries excavation compared with SW (96 % and 91 % compared with 81 % and 61 % after 2 years and 3 years, respectively). Maltz et al. speculated on why stepwise excavation success was only 61 % after 3 years [24]. The authors felt some SW patients did not return for the final excavation and restoration in 1–2 months, and the success rate in these patients was very low (13 %). Patients treated with SW that had a final excavation and permanent restoration had survival rates not statistically different from those of partial excavation (88 % with SW vs. 91 % partial excavation) [24].

4.4.4 No Caries Excavation

The last form of caries treatment has been reported in primary teeth. It involves no drilling or excavation of any caries and would be termed no caries excavation. A steel crown to seal the caries and stop its progress is used [25]. The technique is termed the Hall technique (named after Norma Hall, a Scottish dentist) and presumes that sealing the infected and affected dentin from microleakage will arrest the caries [25, 26]. There have been published reports testing the Hall technique success versus conventional restorations [27, 28]. Ludwig et al. [27] reported in a retrospective study that 65 of 67 steel crowns placed using the Hall technique were successful after a meantime of 15 months. In an RCT report after 12 months, the Hall technique crowns were significantly better ($p=0.002$) than using conventional complete excavation and a compomer restoration [28]. Whether the Hall technique is indicated for use in teeth with deep dentinal caries is yet unknown. In a 10-year prospective study [29], frank carious lesions in permanent teeth that extended radiographically into less than half the dentin were sealed. No caries excavation was done, and the caries was sealed in place with a self-setting occlusal sealant. The report showed arrest of the lesions over 10 years if the occlusal sealant stayed intact. The study's purpose was not intended to promote leaving caries unexcavated, but to show if caries was sealed in place by a sealant, it would not progress [29].

4.5 Indirect Pulp Treatment (IPT)

IPT is a vital pulp treatment where the deepest caries is left unexcavated to avoid causing a pulp exposure due to caries excavation. IPT is indicated for primary and permanent teeth [1]. IPT involves two major suppositions for its success: correctly diagnosing that the pulp is vital and placing a final restoration that prevents microleakage [1, 30]. Reaching the correct pulpal diagnosis in primary teeth will be discussed in detail in Sect. 4.6. Preventing microleakage can be achieved through the use of immediate steel crown placement or a well-bonded composite restoration [31, 32].

4.5.1 Indirect Pulp Treatment Procedure

The IPT procedure is normally done in one appointment but can be done as a modification of the SW procedure in two visits. An IPT begins with removal of the superficial infected dentin using a high-speed water-cooled bur [33]. First, the decay in the periphery of the lesion is excavated completely using slow-speed burs such as #4 or #6. Using the same slow-speed bur, partial excavation of superficial decay on the pulpal floor is done, leaving some decay and not exposing the pulp [33]. Using an excavator for the pulpal floor, excavation may remove large pieces of dentin, which can result in a pulp exposure. The amount of decay remaining appears not to be critical, as dentin remineralization occurs irrespective of the amount of decay remaining [34, 35]. The decay remaining is mostly affected dentin. It may appear moist and soft or dark and leathery, but the dentin color and consistency are not critical to IPT success. If a biological seal is created with a final restoration, the remaining bacteria in the dentin are believed to be nonviable, and the affected dentin will remineralize and become harder [20, 34]. A steel crown or a well-bonded composite resin will prevent any microleakage and maximize the likelihood of success (Fig. 4.7).

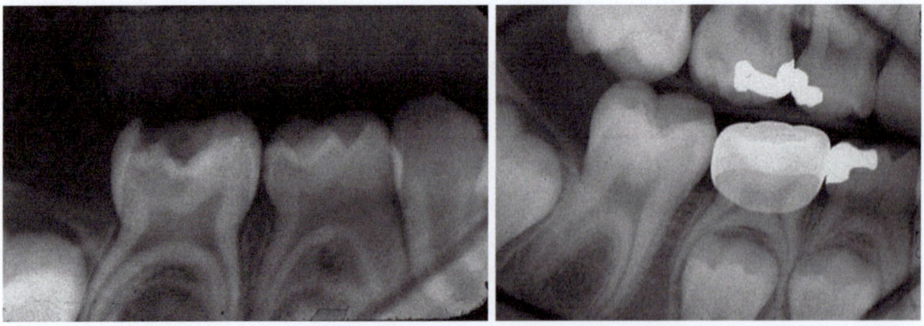

Fig. 4.7 Second primary molar without signs of soft tissue pathology but with a history of pain of short duration when chewing foods (*left*). A one-visit indirect pulp treatment was performed and a steel crown placed to minimize microleakage. Posttreatment radiograph (*right*) 5 years later showing no sign of pathology. The tooth exfoliated normally

4.5.2 Studies on IPT Success

There have been many studies on IPT success. One RCT investigated the success of IPT in primary and permanent molars using a one- and two-visit approach versus complete excavation [36]. This study involved 94 primary second molars and 60 immature permanent first molars with 50 one-visit IPTs, 49 with two-visit IPTs, and 55 done with complete excavation. The IPT base was calcium hydroxide, and the two-visit method used reinforced zinc oxide as a temporary filling over the calcium hydroxide. The primary teeth were restored with a compomer, and the permanent teeth with a bonded composite. There were significantly less pulp exposures with both IPT methods ($p = .008$). The combined IPT groups after 1 year had a success of 91 out of 92 teeth (99 %) that was not statistically different than complete excavation success 41 out of 43 teeth (95 %). Another RCT evaluated IPT in primary molars without a base (bonded composite to the demineralized dentin) versus a calcium hydroxide IPT restored with a bonded composite [37]. The 2-year follow-up of 31 teeth showed an overall success of 87 % with no statistical difference between groups. A third RCT report showed a 94 % success rate of a calcium hydroxide IPT in primary molars after 12–29 months [38]. A longer follow-up period (>3 years) was reported in a retrospective study of 108 IPTs versus 118 formocresol pulpotomies [39]. The IPTs had glass ionomer as a liner. The authors found that after 1 year, the 98 % IPT success was not statistically different from the 95 % pulpotomy success. After the 1–2-year time frame, IPT success was always statistically higher, and the >3-year follow-up showed that IPT success was 94 % while formocresol pulpotomy success was 70 % [39]. All teeth were restored the day of treatment with a steel crown, amalgam, glass ionomer, or composite. It appears from these studies and others [2, 40, 41] that IPT success remains above 80 % no matter the follow-up time, the liner used, and whether it was a one-visit or a two-visit procedure.

There is one unpublished randomized controlled study comparing IPT to a formocresol pulpotomy [42]. The results, after more than 1 year in 26 pairs of primary molars, showed significantly more pathologic radiographic changes in the formocresol pulpotomies than in the IPT group ($p = 0.003$). All teeth were restored with a steel crown.

4.6 Reaching the Correct Pulpal Diagnosis

Correctly diagnosing pulp vitality in primary and immature permanent teeth differs from what is done for a mature permanent tooth [1] (see Chap. 8 for more information on pulpal treatment for the immature permanent tooth). In addition to the history of pain, pulp vitality assessment includes radiographs, a clinical exam, and other adjuncts. Please refer to Chap. 3, Clinical Pulpal Diagnosis, for more information. In children, Coll [2] suggested an adjunct was needed to reliably diagnose pulp vitality with deep caries and proposed using an interim therapeutic restoration (ITR) as the tool.

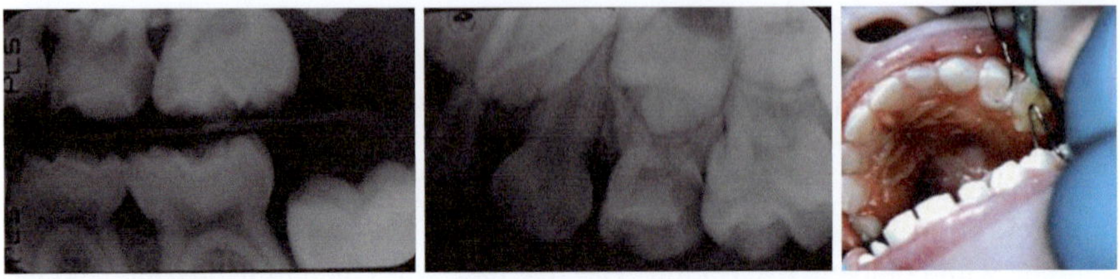

Fig. 4.8 A maxillary left first primary molar with large distal caries that had been causing pain while eating, but without a history of spontaneous unprovoked toothache (*left and center*). A glass ionomer ITR was placed after partial excavation of the lesion to clean out food and some superficial decay to allow space for the ITR (*right*)

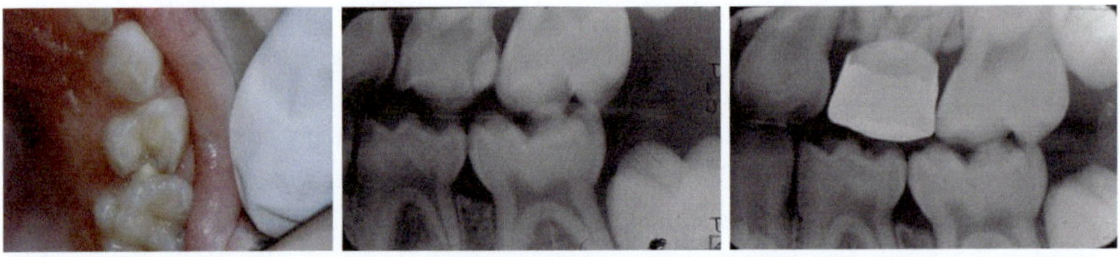

Fig. 4.9 Same first primary molar two months after ITR. The tooth is asymptomatic and demonstrating normal soft tissue (*left*). A radiograph shows that the decay does not reach the pulp (*center*). An indirect pulp treatment was done with an immediate steel crown (*right*). The tooth exfoliated normally

4.6.1 Interim Therapeutic Restoration (ITR) for Pulpal Diagnosis

Coll [2] feels that primary molars with deep caries and an open or closed carious lesion that may exhibit no pain, have elicited pain from chewing foods, or may have questionable spontaneous pain are candidates for using ITR for diagnosis. His retrospective study [2] showed reliable success in diagnosing the vitality of primary molars. The study involved 50 primary molars treated with a glass ionomer ITR for 1–3 months and 63 without an ITR prior to their vital pulp treatment (IPT or formocresol pulpotomy). The ITR procedure was usually done at the initial examination visit. Coll utilized partial caries excavation of the superficial, infected dentin using a spoon excavator or slow-speed round bur (# 4–6), without creating clean margins in the lesion. For a closed lesion, a bur was used to open into the superficial infected dentin to allow an ITR to be inserted. A self-setting glass ionomer ITR was placed without a matrix band. The occlusion was checked with articulating paper (Fig. 4.8).

In the study [2], the patients with an ITR returned 1–3 months later. The soft tissue was inspected for a fistula or swelling, and the parent was questioned if any pain had occurred or if pain had been present, to see if it had stopped. A new radiograph was taken to reassess the tooth (Fig. 4.9). These ITR-treated teeth were diagnosed as vital if there was absence of clinical and radiographic signs and symptoms indicating irreversible pulpitis. Diagnostic success in the ITR-treated teeth and teeth without ITR was based on whether the IPT or vital formocresol pulpotomy succeeded after a meantime of 34.7 months since all teeth had an immediate steel crown placed.

After 34.7 months, Coll [2] found there were three IPT failures in the 53 teeth that received an ITR and were assessed as pulpal diagnostic failures, but the other 50 were assessed as diagnostic successes (94 %). In the 64 teeth not receiving a diagnostic ITR, 14 failed (4 IPT and 10 formocresol pulpotomies) and were assessed as pulpal diagnostic failures leaving 50 diagnostic successes (78 %). The pretreatment ITR significantly improved the ability to correctly make the correct pulpal diagnostic assessment ($P=0.013$). Since all teeth received a steel crown to minimize microleakage, it was assumed any failure of the vital pulp treatment was due to diagnosis. Vital pulp therapy diagnostic success was improved with a diagnostic ITR for 1–3 months if the tooth returned without pain and no signs or symptoms of irreversible pulpitis. Teeth with an ITR diagnosed with irreversible pulpitis returned with pain, soft tissue swelling, or furcation radiolucency on the new radiograph; then no vital pulp treatment was done.

4.7 IPT Liners for Pulpal Floor Bases

The IPT studies cited previously used various liners and/or techniques such as a composite bonded to the dentin [37], calcium hydroxide liner [17, 38, 41], glass ionomer liner [2, 40], and no excavation or liner, just the cement used for the steel crown [26, 27]. Is the liner or what is placed on the pulpal floor critical to IPT success?

Two studies have reported on the effect of the liner over caries [34, 35]. Corralo and Maltz [35] evaluated the effect a liner had on the carious dentin by testing calcium hydroxide, glass ionomer, and a wax liner as a control. Sixty permanent teeth with deep caries had partial caries excavation and one of the liners, and then they were temporized for 3–4 months. The teeth were reopened, and the dentin was clinically assessed (color and consistency) and analyzed for microbial growth.

Irrespective of the dentin liner used, including wax, after 3–4 months, there were dentin hardening, decreased bacterial numbers, and dentin reorganization. Kuhn et al. [34] also studied permanent molars lined with glass ionomer or wax but also analyzed the infected dentin mineral content at 60 days and performed a 10–15-month radiographic follow-up. No caries excavation was done on the pulpal floor before a glass ionomer or wax liner was placed and the tooth restored with composite. After 60 days, the tooth was reopened and a dentin sample taken. The wax was removed if present, and the infected and affected dentin was left in place. All teeth were restored with a bonded composite. Serial radiographs were evaluated to determine if the unexcavated caries remineralized. The results showed increased dentin remineralization and mineral gain after 10–15 months regardless of the liner and the presence of infected dentin. Kuhn et al. [34] felt that sealing the caries from microleakage appears to be the important factor in IPT success, not the liner or technique used if the pulp is correctly diagnosed as vital.

Conclusions

- Complete excavation of the deep carious lesion will cause more pulp exposures compared to stepwise or partial excavation.
- Direct pulp capping after excavating deep caries in primary teeth is contraindicated. Direct pulp capping for pulp exposures caused during deep caries excavation has a low success rate in permanent teeth.
- Stepwise and partial caries excavation done as a one- or two-step IPT has been shown to have high success rates (>80 %) in primary and permanent teeth.
- The use of an interim therapeutic restoration (ITR) at the initial appointment for deep caries for 1–3 months improves the pulpal diagnosis and the success of primary tooth pulp treatment.
- Dentists should not be concerned with the pulpal liner over the caries nor with the amount of decay left in place when doing an IPT, but should be concerned with placing a restoration that stops microleakage.

References

1. AAPD Reference Manual. Guideline on pulp therapy for primary and immature permanent teeth. 2014–2015;36:242–50.
2. Coll JA, Campbell A, Chalmers NI. Effects of glass ionomer temporary restorations on pulpal diagnosis and treatment outcomes in primary molars. Pediatr Dent. 2013;35:416–21.
3. Bergenholtz G, Axelsson S, Davidson T, Frisk F, Hakeberg M, Kvist T, Norlund A, Petersson A, Portenier I, Sandberg H, Tranæus S, Mejare I. Treatment of pulps in teeth affected by deep caries – a systematic review of the literature. Singapore Dent J. 2013;34(1):1–12.
4. Smith AJ, Cassidy N, Perry H, Begue-Kirn C, Ruch JV, Lesot H. Reactionary dentinogenesis. Int J Dev Biol. 1995;39:273–80.
5. Marshall GW, et al. The dentin substrate: structure and properties related to bonding. J Dent. 1997;25:441–58.
6. Fusayama T. Two layers of carious dentin: diagnosis and treatment. Oper Dent. 1979;4:63–70.
7. Bjorndal L. Dentin and pulp reactions to caries and operative treatment: biological variables affecting treatment outcome. Endod Top. 2002;2:10–23.
8. Johnson W, Taylor BR, Berman DS. The response of deciduous dentine to caries studied by correlated light and electron microscopy. Caries Res. 1969;3:348–68.
9. Mjör IA. Dentin-predentin complex and its permeability. Pathology and treatment. Overview. J Dent Res. 1985;64(spec issue):621–7.
10. Edwardsson S. Bacteriology of dentin caries. In: Thylstrup A, Leach SA, Qvist V, editors. Dentine and dentine reactions in the oral cavity. Oxford: IRL Press; 1987. p. 95–102.
11. Kidd EAM, Smith BGN, Pickard HM. Pickard's manual of operative dentistry. 7th ed. Oxford: Oxford University Press; 1998.
12. Schwendicke F, Dörfer CE, Paris S. Incomplete caries removal: a systematic review and meta-analysis. J Dent Res. 2013;92:306–14.
13. Ricketts D, Lamont T, Innes NPT, Kidd E, Clarkson JE. Operative caries management in adults and children. Cochrane Database Syst Rev. 2013;(3):CD003808.
14. Elderton RJ. Clinical studies concerning re-restoration of teeth. Adv Dent Res. 1990;4:4–9.
15. Murray PE, Smith AJ, Windsor LJ, Mjör IA. Remaining dentine thickness and human pulp responses. Int Endod J. 2003;36:33–43.

16. Fuks AB. Pulp therapy for the primary dentition. In: Pinkham JR, Casamassimo PS, Fields Jr HW, McTigue DJ, Nowak A, editors. Pediatric dentistry: infancy through adolescence. 5th ed. St. Louis: Elsevier Saunders Co; 2013. p. 331–51.
17. Bjørndal L, Reit C, Bruun G, Markvart M, Kjældgaard M, Näsman P, et al. Treatment of deep caries lesions in adults: randomized clinical trials comparing stepwise vs. direct complete excavation, and direct pulp capping vs. partial pulpotomy. Eur J Oral Sci. 2010;118:290–7.
18. Al-Hiyasat AS, Barrieshi-Nusair KM, Al-Omari MA. The radiographic outcomes of direct pulp-capping procedures performed by dental students: a retrospective study. J Am Dent Assoc. 2006;137:1699–705.
19. Bogen G, Kim JS, Bakland LK. Direct pulp capping with mineral trioxide aggregate: an observational study. J Am Dent Assoc. 2008;139:305–15.
20. Bjørndal L, Larsen T, Thylstrup A. A clinical and microbiological study of deep carious lesions during stepwise excavation using long treatment intervals. Caries Res. 1997;31: 411–7.
21. Wambier DS, dos Santos FA, Guedes-Pinto AC, Jaeger RG, Simionato MR. Ultrastructural and microbiological analysis of the dentin layers affected by caries lesions in primary molars treated by minimal intervention. Pediatr Dent. 2007;29:228–34.
22. Bjørndal L, Kidd E. The treatment of deep dentine caries lesions. Dent Update. 2005;32: 402–4, 407–10, 413.
23. Maltz M, Moura MS, Jardim JJ, et al. Partial caries removal in deep lesions: 19–30 months follow-up study. Rev Fac Odontol Porto Alegre. 2010;51:20–3.
24. Maltz M, Garcia R, Jardim JJ, de Paula LM, Yamaguti PM, Moura MS, et al. Randomized trial of partial *vs.* stepwise caries removal. J Dent Res. 2012;91:1026–31.
25. Innes NP, Evans DJ, Stirrups DR. The Hall technique; a randomized controlled clinical trial of a novel method of managing carious primary molars in general dental practice: acceptability of the technique and outcomes at 23 months. BMC Oral Health. 2007;7:18.
26. Innes NPT, Evans DJP, Stirrups DR. Sealing caries in primary molars; randomized control trial. 5-year results. J Dent Res. 2011;90:1405–10.
27. Ludwig KH, Fontana M, Vinson LA, Platt JA, Dean JA. The success of stainless steel crowns placed with the Hall technique: a retrospective study. J Am Dent Assoc. 2014;145(12): 1248–53.
28. Santamaria RM, Innes NP, Machiulskiene V, Evans DJ, Splieth CH. Caries management strategies for primary molars: 1-yr randomized control trial results. J Dent Res. 2014;93:1062–9.
29. Mertz-Fairhurst EJ, Curtis JW, Ergle JW, Rueggeberg FA, Adair SM. Ultraconservative and cariostatic sealed restorations: results at year 10. J Am Dent Assoc. 1998;129:55–66.
30. Holan G, Eidelman E, Fuks AB. Long-term evaluation of pulpotomy in primary molars using mineral trioxide aggregate or formocresol. Pediatr Dent. 2005;27:129–36.
31. Hutcheson C, Seale NS, McWhorter A, Kerins C, Wright J. Multi-surface composite vs stainless steel crown restorations after mineral trioxide aggregate pulpotomy: a randomized controlled trial. Pediatr Dent. 2012;34(7):460–7.
32. Guelmann M, Bookmyer KL, Villalta P, García-Godoy F. Microleakage of restorative techniques for pulpotomized primary molars. J Dent Child. 2004;71:209–11.
33. Seale NS, Coll JA. Vital pulp therapy for the primary dentition. Gen Dent. 2010;58(3): 194–200.
34. Kuhn E, Chibinski AC, Reis A, Wambier DS. The role of glass ionomer cement on the remineralization of infected dentin: an in vivo study. Pediatr Dent. 2014;36(4):E118–24.
35. Corralo D, Maltz M. Clinical and ultrastructural effects of different liners/restorative materials on deep carious dentin: a randomized clinical trial. Caries Res. 2013;47:243–50.
36. Orhan AI, Oz FT, Orhan K. Pulp exposure occurrence and outcomes after 1- or 2-visit indirect pulp therapy vs complete caries removal in primary and permanent molars. Pediatr Dent. 2010;32:347–55.
37. Casagrande L, Bento LW, Rerin SO, Lucas Ede R, Dalpian DM, de Araujo FB. In vivo outcomes of indirect pulp treatment using a self-etching primer versus calcium hydroxide over the demineralized dentin in primary molars. J Clin Pediatr Dent. 2008;33:131–5.

38. Trairatvorakul C, Sastararuji T. Indirect pulp treatment vs antibiotic sterilization of deep caries in mandibular primary molars. Int J Paediatr Dent. 2014;24:23–31.
39. Vij R, Coll JA, Shelton P, Farooq NS. Caries control and other variables associated with success of primary molar vital pulp therapy. Pediatr Dent. 2004;26:214–20.
40. Farooq NS, Coll JA, Kuwabara A, Shelton P. Success rates of formocresol pulpotomy and indirect pulp therapy in the treatment of deep dentinal caries in primary teeth. Pediatr Dent. 2000;22:278–86.
41. Al-Zayer MA, Straffon LH, Feigal RJ, Welch KB. Indirect pulp treatment of primary posterior teeth: a retrospective study. Pediatr Dent. 2003;25:29–36.
42. Roberts J. Indirect pulp treatment vs. Formocresol pulpotomy in human primary molars: a randomized controlled trial. A thesis. The Texas A&M University System Health Science Center. 2009. Accessed at http://pqdtopen.proquest.com on 8 Aug 2015.

Pulpotomy Techniques: Cervical (Traditional) and Partial

5

Kaaren G. Vargas, Anna B. Fuks, and Benjamin Peretz

Contents

K.G. Vargas, DDS, PhD (✉)
Private Practice Iowa USA, 1738 Lininger Ln, North Liberty, IA 52317, USA
e-mail: kvargas@corridorkidsdentistry.com

A.B. Fuks, DDS
Department of Pediatric Dentistry, Hebrew University, Hadassah School of Dental Medicine, 12272, Jerusalem, Israel
e-mail: fuks@mail.huji.ac.il

B. Peretz, DMD
Department of Pediatric Dentistry, The Maurice and Gabriela Goldschleger School of Dental Medicine, Tel Aviv, Israel
e-mail: bperetz@post.tau.ac.il

A.B. Fuks, B. Peretz (eds.), *Pediatric Endodontics: Current Concepts in Pulp Therapy for Primary and Young Permanent Teeth*,
DOI 10.1007/978-3-319-27553-6_5

5.1 Introduction

The conservation of primary teeth in form and function until their normal exfoliation is one of the fundamental objectives of pediatric dentistry. Not only is it important for normal speech, development, and self-esteem, it is the best way to preserve arch length and avoid secondary issues such as space loss and permanent tooth impaction.

In asymptomatic primary teeth with deep carious lesions approximating the pulp, the coronal pulpotomy is one of the most common ways of achieving the goal of tooth preservation. The objective of the pulpotomy technique is to remove the affected coronal pulp tissue so that the unaffected radicular pulp tissue can continue to function normally until the tooth is ready to exfoliate naturally.

Historically, medicaments that were first used to try and conserve the affected primary tooth in situ had the objective of mummification of the remaining pulp. Over time and with continued research, new products have been tested, both in vitro and in vivo, with outcomes differing from mummification. These new methods have allowed to classify pulpotomy techniques according to the objective of treatment with these different materials.

In today's world of conservative dentistry, we would be remiss if we did not include techniques that do not invade the pulp space or minimally invade the space but have the objective of maintaining pulp vitality in its entirety allowing the tooth to heal. Such are indirect pulp treatment (IPT), as well as those techniques that only partially remove the affected tissue like partial pulpotomy.

Therefore, this chapter will list and discuss the pulpotomy medicaments that have had the most clinical or laboratory trials as well as the respective clinical techniques. In addition, some of the more conservative applications in the context of case selection and diagnosis will be elaborated.

5.2 The Importance of Diagnosis and Evaluation Prior to Treatment Selection

In deep carious lesions or lesions that approximate the pulp, conventional dentistry follows the principles of GV Black of extension for prevention and complete caries excavation. Black stated: "The deeper portion should be freed of any remaining softened material with spoon excavators. In no case should any decayed and softened material be left. It is better to expose the pulp of the tooth than to leave it covered only with softened dentin" [1].

In the latter part of the twentieth century, conservative or minimally invasive dentistry (MID) has revolutionized the approach to caries excavation and diagnosis both in primary and permanent teeth [2]. Leaving affected dentin is acceptable, and where a pulpotomy was most commonly the end result of deep caries in a primary molar or incisor because "pink" could be seen, presently several options to preserve tooth vitality and integrity are available.

Indirect pulp therapy (IPT) is advocated for teeth that are symptomless and have caries approximating the pulp. The outer layers of infected dentin are removed from the walls and floor while leaving affected dentin close to the pulp. Success rates of over 90 % have been reported using this technique under the correct diagnostic conditions [3, 4].

Chapters 3 and 4 of this book are dedicated to an in-depth understanding of both diagnosis and methods of indirect or direct pulp treatment. It is mentioned here because of how much the world of restorative dentistry and pulp therapy is changing and how much this change affects the decision making in treating primary tooth pulp. Adequately distinguishing between an unaffected and an affected dentin-pulp complex is needed to make sound treatment decisions in our effort to preserve the primary tooth until it naturally exfoliates. Although this chapter is mainly dedicated to pulpotomy techniques, the decisions that should be made are between IPT and pulpectomy, as an unaffected pulp may not require pulp therapy and an infected or affected pulp may benefit more from a pulpectomy than from a pulpotomy.

5.3 Pulpotomy Technique for Primary Teeth

Numerous pulpotomy materials are available to maintain the vitality of the primary radicular pulp aiming to preserve the primary molar in the dental arch. However, there is in essence only one pulpotomy technique prior to medicament placement:

1. Select the tooth to receive the pulp therapy using criteria addressed in Chaps. 3 and 4 of this book. In summary, the tooth should be devoid of spontaneous pain, have no parulis or mobility, and demonstrate no radiographic internal or external root resorption nor furcation radiolucency.
2. Anesthetize using the technique of choice and isolate the tooth preferably with a rubber dam to avoid contamination of the pulp chamber with salivary bacteria (Fig. 5.1).
3. Remove all caries prior to entering the pulp chamber.
4. Once all caries is removed, a #330 carbide bur under copious water spray is used to expose the pulp chamber (Fig. 5.2).

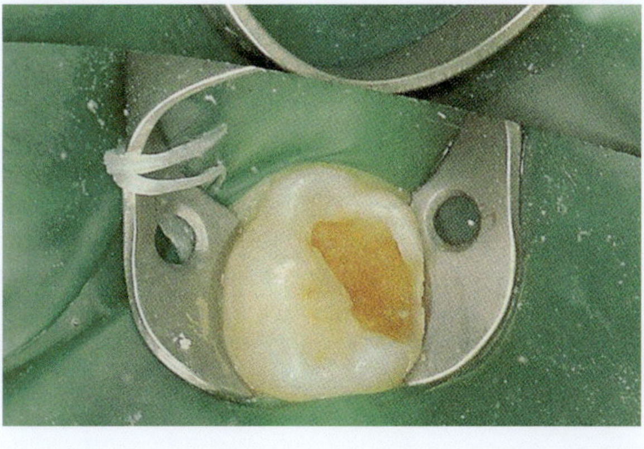

Fig. 5.1 Tooth isolated with a rubber dam prior to caries removal

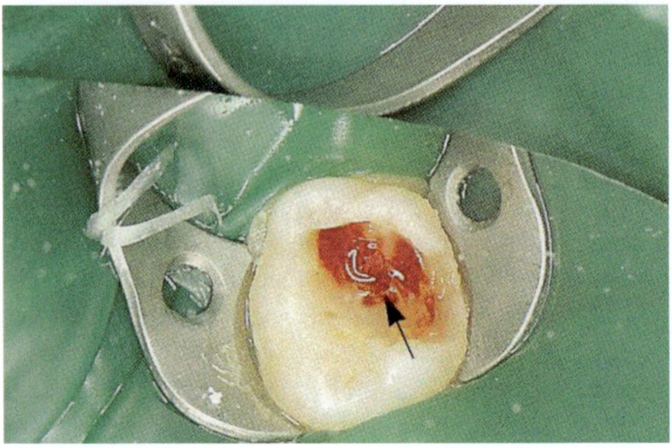

Fig. 5.2 Pulp exposed prior to de-roofing the pulp chamber

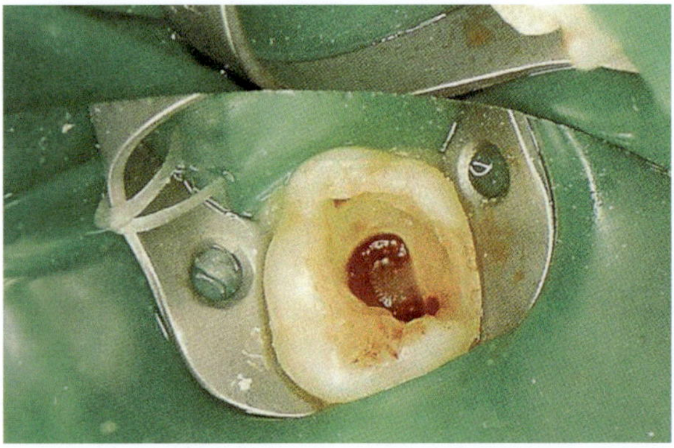

Fig. 5.3 Root canal orifices showing vital tissue after hemostasis

5. Coronal pulp is removed with a round bur on a slow speed handpiece, and hemostasis is achieved by the application of a cotton pellet for no more than 5 min (Fig. 5.3). If hemostasis cannot be achieved, pulpotomy is no longer indicated as the pulp tissue is inflamed and hyperemic. In such condition, an alternative treatment would be needed (pulpectomy or even extraction).
6. Once hemostasis is obtained, the chosen material is placed and the tooth is restored.

5.4 Pulpotomy Materials

Ideally, a pulpotomy medicament should be bactericidal, easy to use, harmless to the remaining pulp tissue and the surrounding structures, should not interfere with physiologic root resorption, and should be relatively inexpensive [5]. Needless to say, the ideal dressing material has not been found, and studies are constantly being conducted in both endodontics and pediatric dentistry to find such a product.

The search for this ideal material has been ongoing since the early 1900s when Buckley first introduced formocresol [6]. Over the years, many other materials have surfaced as potential candidates and have been classified into three major categories according to their effects on the remaining radicular pulp.

5.5 Classification of Vital Pulp Therapy

Types	Other name
Devitalizing	Mummification; cauterization
Preserving	Minimal devitalization; noninducive
Regenerating	Inductive; reparative

Some of the seminal studies for each method can be summarized in the following table taken from Ranly, 1994, and modified [7].

Timeline	Devitalizing	Preserving	Regenerating
1930	Multiple Visits with Formocresol [9]		
1938			CaOH Pulpotomy for Primary Teeth (Teuscher and Zander 1938)
1962	*2 Visit FC Pulpotomy* Human [8]		
1965	*5 min FC Pulpotomy* Animal (Spedding et al. 1965)		
1966	Human (Redig 1966)		
1970	*Dilution of FC Animal* (Straffon and Han 1970)		CaOH Evaluated Human [40]
1971	[12]	ZOE Evaluated Human (Magnusson 1971) Ledermix Introduced Human (Hansen et al. 1971)	
1975	Dilution of FC; Human (Morawa 1975)	Glutaraldeyde Proposed RCT (s-Gravenmande 1975)	
1978	Systemic Distribution of FC Animal [15]	Glutaraldeyde Proposed Pulpotomy (Ranly and Lazzari 1978)	
1980		GA Proposed Humans (Kopel 1980)	
1981	Dilution of FC (Omission from ZOE) Animal (Garcia-Godoy 1981)		
1983	Systemic Effects Animal (Myers et al. 1983) Electrosurgical Pulpotomy animal (Ruemping et al. 1983)		

(continued)

Table (continued)

Timeline	Devitalizing	Preserving	Regenerating
1984			Enriched Collagen (Fuks 1984) Hard Setting CaOH (Heilig 1984)
1985	Laser animal (Shoji et al. 1985)		
1988			Freeze Dried Bone (Fadavi et al. 1988)
1989			Demineralized Dentin (Nakashima 1989)
1991		Ferric Sulfate Human (Fei 1991)	Bone Morphogenetic Protein Animal (Nakashima 1991)
1993	Electrosurgical Pulpotomy Human (Mack 1993)		Osteogenic Protein (Rutherford 1993)
1996	Argon Laser Animal (Wilkerson 1996)		MTA Animal (Ford et al. 1996)
2001			MTA Human (Eidelman et al. 2001)
2002		Sodium Hypochlorite Animal (Hafez et al. 2002)	
2006		Sodium Hypochlorite Human [31]	

Thus, there have been numerous pulp dressing materials tested over the decades with varying success. This chapter will focus on the most common, most studied, and most successful representatives of each materials.

5.6 Devitalizing

The Webster dictionary defines "devitalize" as means to deprive of vitality or vital properties, make lifeless, to weaken (merriem-webster.com/dictionary/devitalize). These products are designed to mummify the remaining pulp tissue and are represented by formocresol, laser, and electro surgery. As the most universally accepted method, formocresol will be discussed.

5.6.1 Formocresol

Formocresol was first introduced by Buckley as a treatment of non-vital permanent teeth in 1904 [6, 8] and consisted of equal parts of formalin and cresol. It was not until 1930, however, that formocresol was introduced as a pulpotomy medicament for non-vital primary teeth with the formulation of 19 % formaldehyde and 35 % cresol in a vehicle of glycerin or water [7, 9].

A multistep process of four visits was proposed for mummifying the radicular pulp tissue completely, thereby eliminating the likelihood of internal resorption [7]. Microscopic analysis by Emmerson et al. showed that most of the beneficial effects of formocresol was in the first 5 min; moreover, they showed that prolonged exposure caused calcific degeneration [10]. Thus, the original four-visit technique was revised to the currently accepted one-visit, 5-min-application, as introduced by Redig in 1968 [11].

Although this method of application saved time, it rendered the pulp tissue only partially vital leaving the tissue susceptible to abscess formation and/or internal root resorption [11]. In 1971, Loos and Han evaluated the effects of different concentrations of formocresol and found that a 1:5 dilution was as effective as the full strength [12].

Rolling and Lambjerg-Hansen studied histologically teeth that had been successfully treated with formocresol and observed that the remaining radicular pulps had severe inflammation adjacent to the amputation site, and most had areas of necrosis within the remaining pulp tissue without evidence of pulp fixation [13]. From these observations, the authors concluded that the formocresol option should be reserved as a means to keep the affected primary teeth functioning for a limited period of time. Regardless of this outcome, it has been the benchmark against which all other pulpotomy medicaments are measured.

Numerous studies have been conducted since the 1930s and have found success rates varying from 55 to 95 % [7]. These rates vary based on the type of study, criteria for success, and the follow-up period.

Over the years, formocresol has been labeled as being mutagenic, toxic, and carcinogenic [14–16]. However, little to no evidence actually exists to implicate formocresol in any of these allegations [17]. Regardless, the gavel has been swung, the verdict has been delivered, and formocresol as a pulpotomy medicament is becoming less popular. To further compound the issue, the International Agency for Research on Cancer classified formaldehyde as carcinogenic for humans in June 2004 [50]. With this new classification, the need to assess new materials to replace the long-standing formocresol has become crucial.

5.6.1.1 Formocresol Pulpotomy Technique

1. Once the pulp tissue has been removed from the pulp chamber and bleeding has been controlled, a cotton pellet dipped in a 1:5 dilution of the original Buckley's formocresol and the excess are expressed to ensure very little moisture on the cotton pellet (Fig. 5.4).
2. The dampened cotton pellet is applied in the pulp chamber for 5 min (Fig. 5.5).
3. The cotton pellet is removed, and the root canal orifices are expected to look like "black eyes", with no bleeding. The pulp chamber is then filled with a thick paste of zinc oxide eugenol (ZOE) or intermediate restorative material (IRM) (Fig. 5.6), and the tooth is restored with the material of choice depending on remaining tooth structure.

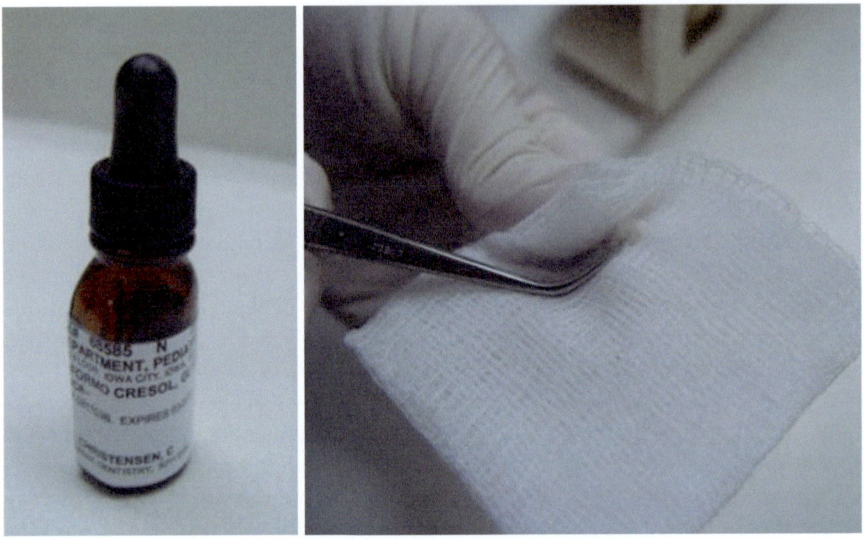

Fig. 5.4 Expressing excess of formocresol (*right*)

Fig. 5.5 Cotton pellet in pulp chamber

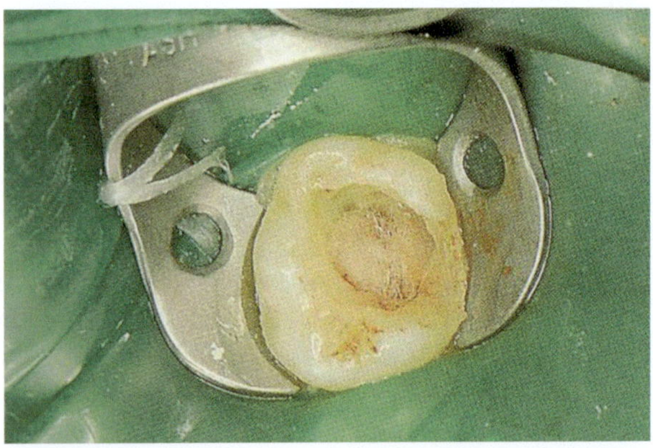

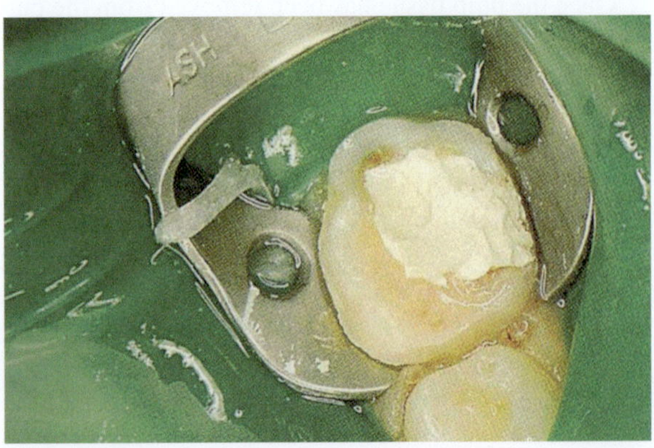

Fig. 5.6 IRM in chamber

5.7 Preserving

By definition, preserving means to keep from injury, peril, harm; to protect. Therefore, the objective of the materials included in this category is to minimally insult the tissue in order to preserve the vitality of the radicular pulp [7]. As representatives of this category, glutaraldehyde, ferric sulfate, and sodium hypochlorite (NaOCl) will be discussed.

5.7.1 Glutaraldehyde

Glutaraldehyde is a colorless, oily liquid that is used as an antimicrobial agent in water treatment lines, a preservative in cosmetics, and as a cold sterilizing material in the healthcare industry (http://www.cdc.gov/niosh/topics/glutaraldehyde/).

Glutaraldehyde is a di-aldehyde that has superior fixative properties over formocresol and has self-limiting penetration, low antigenicity, low toxicity, and eliminates cresol. Glutaraldehyde has no bactericidal ability at low pH and therefore must be alkalinized to a pH of between 7.5 and 8.5 before it is effective. This increase in pH renders glutaraldehyde unstable, thus decreasing its shelf life to approximately 14 days [18]. Some formulations increase the life of this product to 1 or 2 weeks [18].

s-Gravenmade [19] proposed glutaraldehyde as an alternative to formocresol in endodontic procedures in 1975. He observed that, unlike formocresol, glutaraldehyde did not diffuse laterally or apically through the root length, making it a safer alternative to formocresol.

In 1980, Kopel et al. introduced glutaraldehyde into primary tooth pulpotomies as an attempt to find a material that was less toxic than formocresol, was self-limiting, and preserved the radicular pulp [20]. The authors used a 2 % glutaraldehyde solution over the amputated pulp stumps and then incorporated a drop of glutaraldehyde into the ZOE paste which was placed in the pulp chamber. Garcia-Godoy et al. used a 2 % formulation with similar findings [21]. The clinical and histological findings of both these studies prompted the proposal that glutaraldehyde was a viable alternative to formocresol as a pulpotomy medicament for primary teeth. The results of a study by Fuks et al. were not so promising and perhaps slowed down the impact that glutaraldehyde was gaining [22, 23].

Histologically, glutaraldehyde is a better fixative at higher concentrations and longer exposure times than formocresol, yet demonstrates less penetration into the subsurfaces, leading to less formation of zones of necrosis and granulation tissue [24]. Lloyd et al. studied various concentrations of glutaraldehyde over differing times in primates and found that the effectiveness of glutaraldehyde was inversely proportional to both the concentration and length of the exposure. The lower the concentration, the longer the glutaraldehyde needed to be in contact with the remaining radicular pulp for effectiveness to be maintained. Their results showed a concentration of 2 % with an exposure time of 10 min to have the most favorable success over time [25].

Several human studies have shown success rates ranging from 82 to 95 % [7], yet, perhaps due to its instability and short life span, glutaraldehyde has not gained the popularity that other materials in this category have.

5.7.1.1 Glutaraldehyde Pulpotomy Technique

The glutaraldehyde pulpotomy technique is identical to the formocresol pulpotomy technique with the exception that the solution on the cotton pellet is not expressed. Studies have shown variation in success based on the relative wetness of the cotton pellet [25]. The recommendation currently is to have the cotton pellet soaked in glutaraldehyde and applied very wet.

5.7.2 Ferric Sulfate

Ferric sulfate is an agglutinating agent thought to produce hemostasis by blood reaction with both the ferric and sulfate ions as well as with the acidic pH of the solution [26]. The hemostasis achieved by this agglutination is thought to reduce the likelihood of clot breakdown and subsequent inflammatory response [27].

It has been shown that the application of ferric sulfate prior to calcium hydroxide in pulpotomized primate teeth had more favorable results than calcium hydroxide alone [28]. Similarly, Fei et al. compared ferric sulfate to formocresol in a 12-month clinical trial and found that ferric sulfate had better success than formocresol [29]. Since then, numerous studies have been done comparing ferric sulfate to a number of materials including formocresol with differing results.

Histologically, Fuks et al. showed that like formocresol, ferric sulfate does not promote healing of the remaining pulp tissue, and there are several degrees of chronic inflammation [26].

The most common controversy concerning the use of ferric sulfate has been the radiographic appearance of significant internal resorption (Fig. 5.7) leading to premature exfoliation [30]. This could be an issue if the pulpotomy is performed on a very young child where tooth retention is of utmost importance. Nevertheless, both the favorable results and the ease of use of the 15.5 % solution have propelled this technique into one of the most popular alternatives to formocresol.

5.7.2.1 Internal Resorption Associated with Ferric Sulfate

Ferric Sulfate Pulpotomy Technique

1. Once the pulp chamber is accessed, the coronal pulp is removed and gross hemostasis is achieved with a cotton pellet.
2. A 15.5 % ferric sulfate solution is applied to the pulp stumps until complete hemostasis is present. Notice the typical dark appearance of the tissue affected by the ferric sulfate (Fig. 5.8).
3. A thick paste of ZOE or IRM is placed in the chamber and tooth is restored (Fig. 5.9).

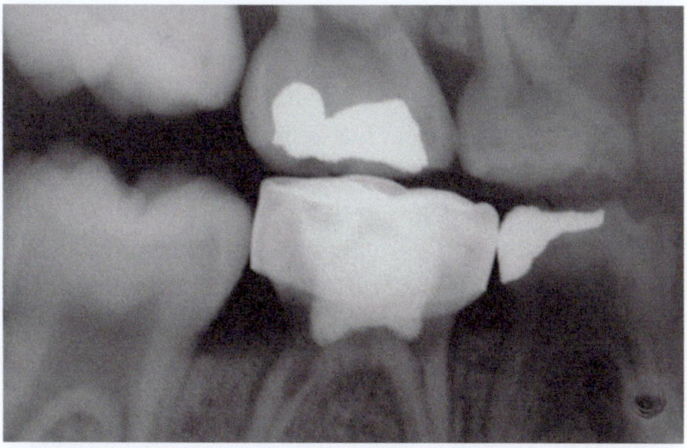

Fig. 5.7 Note internal resorption in tooth 85 (T) 6 months after a ferric sulfate pulpotomy was performed [31]

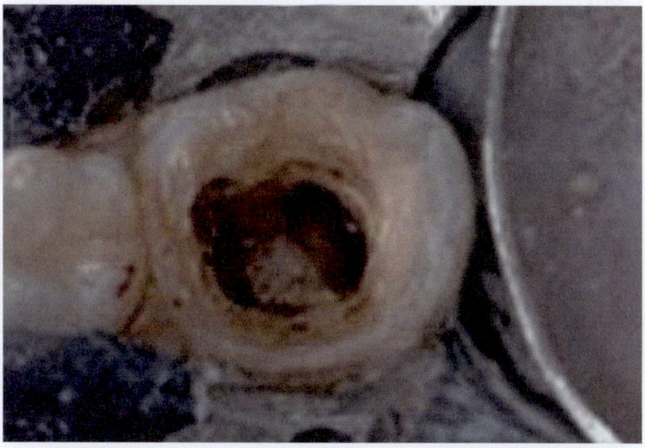

Fig. 5.8 Dark appearance of tissue after application of ferric sulfate

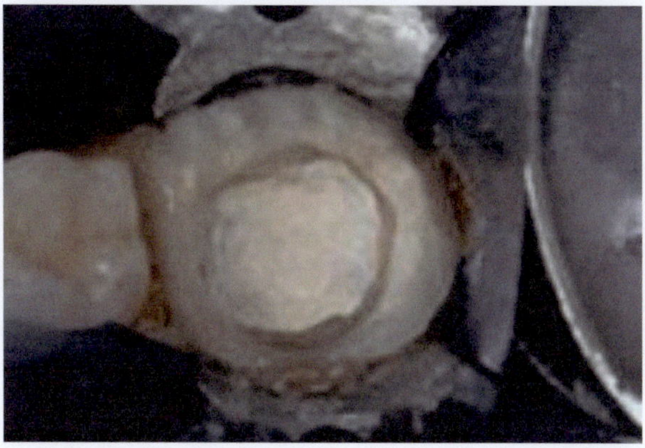

Fig. 5.9 Placement of IRM in pulp chamber

5.7.3 Sodium Hypochlorite

Sodium hypochlorite (NaOCl) has been used as a root canal irrigant for permanent teeth since the 1920s and has been shown to be a very good antibacterial agent without being a significant irritant to the pulp tissue [31].

Rosenfeld et al. showed that placement of 5 % NaOCl on non-instrumented vital pulp tissue acted only at the surface, with minimal effects on deeper pulpal tissue [32]. Hafez et al. showed no pulpal inflammation after bleeding control was obtained with 3 % NaOCl in pulpotomized adult monkey teeth [33, 34]. Accorinte et al. evaluated $FeSO_4$, NaOCl, calcium hydroxide ($Ca(OH)_2$), and saline as hemostatic agents in pulpotomized human premolars restored with adhesive and composite resin. Their results showed that 60 % of the subjects with $FeSO_4$ pulpotomies had sensitivity to cold, and histological analysis showed intense inflammatory response. Conversely, none of the patients treated with NaOCl or $Ca(OH)_2$ reported any pain or sensitivity. Histological assessment also showed comparable chronic inflammation for both of these medicaments [35].

Vargas et al. conducted a randomized clinical trial (RCT) comparing ferric sulfate to NaOCl and found an overall success rate of 90 % over a 12-month period compared to a 74 % success rate for ferric sulfate [31]. Since then three other RCTs have been conducted to evaluate the success of 3–5 % solutions of NaOCl with similar results to both formocresol and ferric sulfate [35–38].

Histologically, NaOCl is compatible with pulp tissue and has only superficial effects on vital pulp tissue [32].

5.7.3.1 Sodium Hypochlorite Pulpotomy Technique

1. Once the pulp chamber is accessed, the coronal pulp is removed and hemostasis is achieved with a cotton pellet.
2. A cotton pellet is moistened in 3 % or 5 % NaOCl and placed in the chamber for 30 s.
3. The pellet is removed, the chamber is gently irrigated ensuring no clot is present.
4. ZOE or IRM is placed in the pulp chamber and the tooth is restored.

5.8 Regenerating

By definition, to regenerate is to revive or produce anew; bring into existence again. Thus, by definition, the pulpotomy medicament in this category should be one that leaves the remaining radicular pulp vital and completely enclosed away from the potentially noxious effects of restorative materials and bases.

Materials that belong to this category of pulpotomy medicaments can induce reparative dentin, and their application has been based on sound biologic principles. Representatives of this category are calcium hydroxide ($CaOH_2$) and mineral trioxide aggregate (MTA).

5.8.1 Calcium Hydroxide

Calcium hydroxide ($CaOH_2$) was first introduced by Zander in the 1930s and was thought to have its effects through the modification of a solubility product of Ca and PO_4 and a precipitation of salt into an organic matrix [39]. It is, however, the effect of the very high pH of $CaOH_2$ that most likely initiates either the reparative dentin cascade or one of inflammatory response [7].

From the start, pulpotomies with $CaOH_2$ were fraught with failures; Doyle et al. found a radiographic failure rate of 64 % over 18 months when compared to formocresol [8]. Studies have shown success rates from 31 to 100 % with the majority of failures attributed to internal resorption [40–42].

Perhaps the dismal results shown for calcium hydroxide as a pulpotomy medicament in primary tooth pulpotomies may be due to the chronic inflammation that may already be present. This chronic inflammation or the presence of a blood clot may inhibit the beneficial effects of $CaOH_2$ on the remaining pulp tissue and adversely affect the results [43]. It is also speculated that the high pH of calcium hydroxide wounds the pulp in a manner that initiates the inflammatory cascade [18]. Regardless of what mechanism is activated, the poor success rate of $CaOH_2$ pulpotomies definitely limits its usefulness as a pulpotomy medicament in primary teeth.

5.8.1.1 Calcium Hydroxide Pulpotomy Technique

1. As with all of the pulpotomy techniques, the pulp chamber is de-roofed and hemostasis is obtained with a dry or damp cotton pellet (Fig. 5.10).
2. Once hemostasis is achieved, a $CaOH_2$ paste is placed in the pulp chamber.
3. ZOE or IRM is placed over the $CaOH_2$ and the tooth is restored.

5.8.2 Mineral Trioxide Aggregate (MTA)

Since its introduction into dentistry in 1993, MTA has taken the endodontic world by storm.

MTA is a powder consisting of fine hydrophilic particles that set in the presence of moisture. MTA material is a mixture of a refined Portland cement and bismuth oxide. It contains dicalcium silicate, tricalcium silicate, tricalcium aluminate, and tetracalcium aluminoferrite. It is also reported to contain small amounts of other mineral oxides such as SiO_2, CaO_2, MgO, K_2SO_4, and Na_2SO_4, which modify its chemical and physical properties [44, 45]. MTA has a pH of 12.5 after setting mostly due to the fact that the reaction product of MTA and water is $CaOH_2$ [46].

Subsequent to the report of Torabinejad et al. on root-end sealing materials in 1993 [46], Eidelman et al. showed 100 % success after 17 months with MTA as a vital pulpotomy material [47]. Since then, a large number of articles have been published in the pediatric dentistry literature dealing with pulp therapy and MTA. The results of all these studies show consistent success with very little

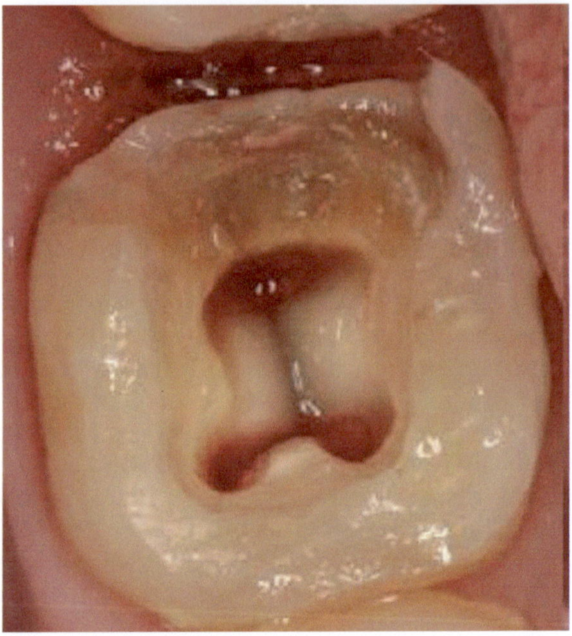

Fig. 5.10 Hemostasis obtained after placement of a dry cotton pellet

adverse events rendering MTA as, perhaps, the most exciting new pulp therapy material in decades.

One of the downsides of MTA is that the presence of iron renders the tooth a dark gray color. Recently white MTA that was supposed to reduce or eliminate the discoloration became available on the market. The results have been slightly inferior to those with gray MTA, and discoloration was still present. Another issue that has to be dealt with especially in the realm of pediatric dentistry is the cost of MTA.

In primary teeth, MTA is predominantly used for direct pulp capping and pulpotomy procedures. The major benefits of MTA are that it is biocompatible, it is bactericidal (high pH, 12.5), and it is able to stimulate cementum-like formation, osteoblastic adherence, and bone regeneration (see Chap. 2). Moreover, its sealing, mineralizing, dentinogenic, and osteogenic potentials make it the preferred choice for numerous clinical applications [48]. Success rates for MTA have ranged from 66 to 100 %, and results have not been too far different from those obtained with formocresol, ferric sulfate, or $NAOCl_2$ [18].

5.8.2.1 MTA Pulpotomy Technique

1. Once the pulp chamber is accessed, the coronal pulp is removed and hemostasis is achieved with a cotton pellet.
2. A 3:1 MTA to sterile saline is mixed into a paste and applied to the pulpal floor (Figs. 5.11 and 5.12).
3. ZOE or IRM is placed over the MTA and the tooth is restored.

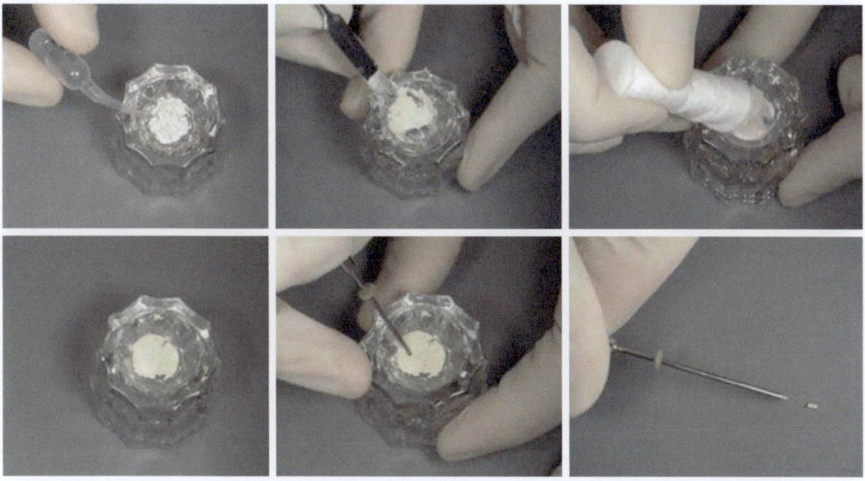

Fig. 5.11 From *upper left*: MTA mix and consistency of final product for placement in pulp chamber

Fig. 5.12 MTA in pulp chamber

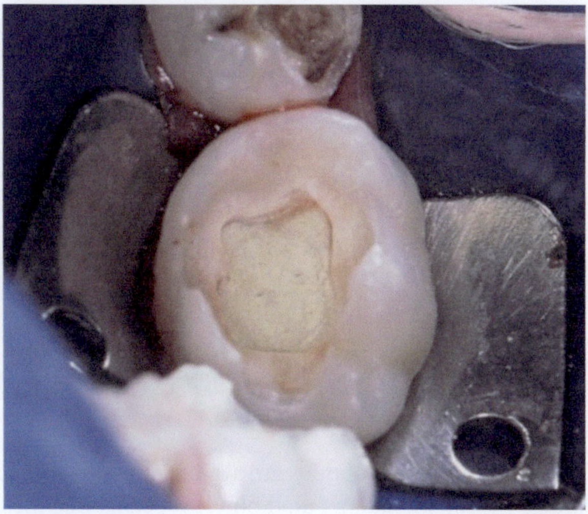

5.9 Partial Pulpotomy Secondary to Trauma or Non-caries-Associated Resorption

Because of the resilience of the supporting structures, trauma to primary incisors is frequently a luxation injury. However, in a few instances, there may be a fracture of the crown, with or without pulp exposure [54]. Unlike pulp exposures due to caries, the pulp in traumatically exposed primary teeth is healthy since it was exposed due to the trauma and not to demineralization caused by bacterial contamination.

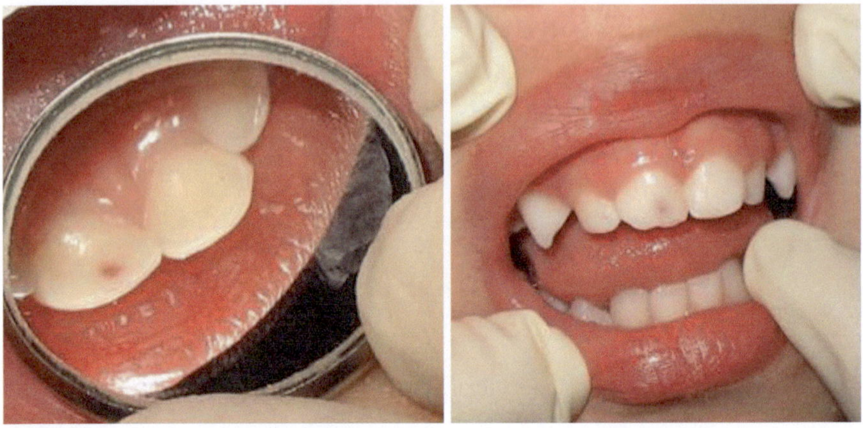

Fig. 5.13 Palatal view (*left*) and facial view (*right*) of the pink area of a possible idiopathic internal resorption. The pulp is not exposed

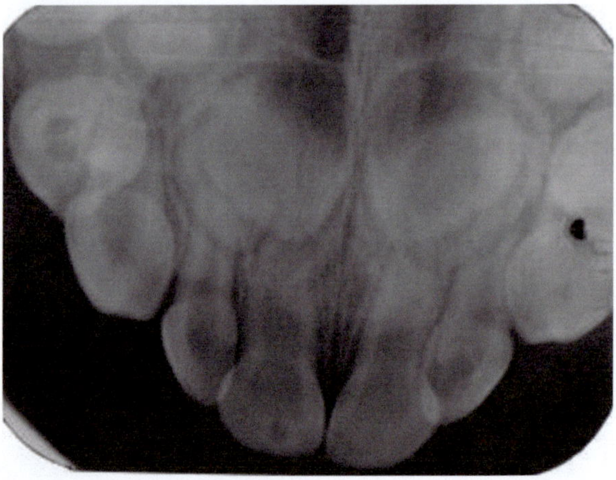

Fig. 5.14 Radiograph of the "pink tooth" showing a radiolucent area at the incisal edge resembling a crack almost reaching the pulp area

Several treatment options are available for crown fractures with pulp exposure in primary teeth, including pulpotomy, root canal treatment, or extraction. The vitality of the tissue and the time elapsed since the injury dictates the treatment of choice. If the pulp tissue is vital, a cervical pulpotomy has been recommended [53]. Cvek advocated the use of a partial pulpotomy which involved the excision of 1–2 mm of the pulp tissue adjacent to the exposure site resulting in the removal of the infected pulp, allowing the application of $CaOH_2$ on healthy tissue [51, 52]. MTA may also be a viable alternative, but one must be cautious with its use as staining of the cervical margin may be a cosmetic issue.

An interesting consideration in cases of primary tooth trauma with pulp exposure or idiopathic internal resorption (Figs. 5.13 and 5.14) may be the partial pulpotomy. Over the years, the treatment of carious exposures of primary teeth with $CaOH_2$

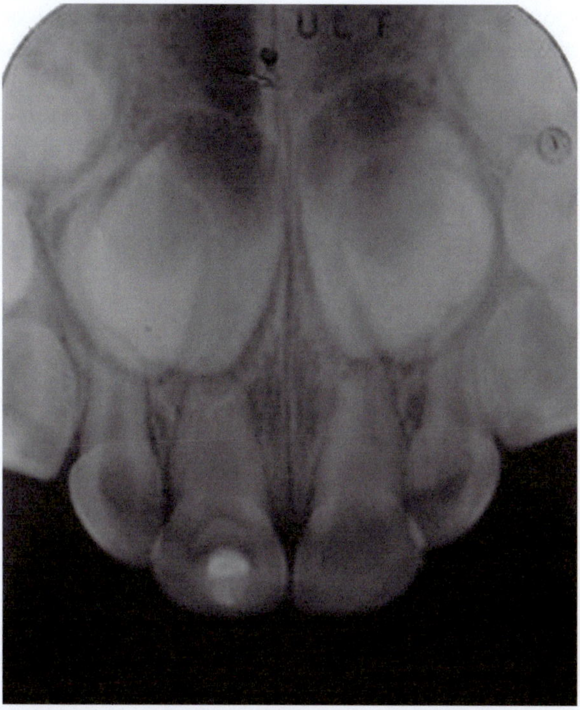

Fig. 5.15 A 2-year result showing a dentin bridge under the pulpotomy area and a vital pulp

partial pulpotomies has had very little success and as a technique is not advocated. It has been shown that $CaOH_2$ has no beneficial effect on inflamed pulps [54]. However, under "sterile" conditions, the use of partial pulpotomy is something that may need to be reconsidered as a possible treatment alternative [55]. The authors suggested performing partial pulpotomy to preserve pulp vitality in a young primary tooth with a wide open apex and thin root dentin walls (Fig. 5.15).

Petel and Fuks (personal communication) have reported the use of this technique for the resolution of idiopathic internal resorption [56].

5.10 Summary

This chapter has presented a number of materials that have been used as pulpotomy medicaments since the early 1900s, as well as alternative thinking and revisiting of old techniques in a new context.

A recent Cochrane Review of pulpotomy medicaments showed that none of the materials was significantly superior, although the trend was for better results with MTA and ferric sulfate [49].

It is possible that the reason why pulpotomies do not present 100 % success may be due to inadequate case selection. If the pulp tissue is truly unaffected or minimally affected, then there should be no reason why pulp treatment should fail. One should always keep in mind that bleeding status may or may not be a true indicator of pulp status. In case of a carious exposure, one can assume that the radicular pulp may have also been adversely affected. The decision may have to be to perform a pulpectomy instead of a pulpotomy, since the radicular pulp may have already begun a process of degeneration, or to perform a pulpotomy with an expected less favorable prognosis.

Therefore, clinically, one should take into consideration numerous factors before deciding what treatment to perform. These factors include:

1. Pulp status
2. Extent of the carious lesion
3. Age of the patient at the time of treatment
4. Goals of the treatment
5. Cost of the treatment

If the child is very young and there is a carious exposure, a pulpectomy may be the treatment of choice. Conversely in an older child with a similar carious exposure, where no long-term maintenance is needed, a pulpotomy may be adequate with any of the materials discussed.

In asymptomatic carious teeth where the lesion radiographically appears close but not overlapping with the pulp space, or in cases when a clear barrier between the caries and the pulp is evident, an indirect pulp treatment (IPT) may be the recommended technique regardless of the age of the child.

Diagnosis is the key to the success of any of these materials and techniques and should always be at the forefront of our thought process when making any decision on pulp therapy.

References

1. Bjorndal L. The caries process and its effect on the pulp: the science is changing and so is our understanding. Pediatr Dent. 2008;30:192–6.
2. Mount GJ. A new paradigm for operative dentistry. Aust Dent J. 2007;52:264–70; quiz 342.
3. Vij R, Coll JA, Shelton P, Farooq NS. Caries control and other variables associated with success of primary molar vital pulp therapy. Pediatr Dent. 2004;26(3):214–20.
4. Al-Zayer MA, Straffon LH, Feigal RJ, Welch KB. Indirect pulp treatment of primary posterior teeth: a retrospective study. Pediatr Dent. 2003;25(1):29–36.
5. Fuks AB, Kupietzki A, Guelmann M. Pulp therapy for the primary dentition. In: infancy through adolescence. In: Casamassimo PS, Fields Jr HW, McTigue DJ, Nowak AJ, editors. Pediatric dentistry: infancy through adolescence. 5th ed. St. Louis: Elsevier Saunders; 2015. p. 333–51.
6. Buckley JP. The chemistry of pulp decomposition with a rational treatment for this condition and its sequelae. Am Dent J. 1904;3:764–71.
7. Ranly DM. Pulpotomy therapy in primary teeth: new modalities for old rationales. Pediat Dent. 1994;16:403–9.
8. Doyle WA, McDonald RE, Mitchell DF. Formocresol versus calcium hydroxide in pulpotomy. ASDC J Dent Child. 1962;29:86–97.
9. Sweet Jr CA. Procedure for treatment of exposed and pulpless deciduous teeth. J Am Dent Assoc. 1930;17:1150–3.

10. Emmerson CC, Miyamoto O, Sweet Sr CA, Bhatia HL. Pulpal changes following formocresol applications on rat molars and human primary teeth. J Cal Dent Assoc. 1959;27:309–23.
11. Redig DF. A comparison and evaluation of two formocresol pulpotomy technics utilizing "Buckley's" formocresol. J Dent Child. 1968;35(1):22–30.
12. Loos PJ, Han SS. An enzyme histochemical study of the effect of various concentrations of formocresol on connective tissues. Oral Surg Oral Med Oral Path. 1971;31(4):571–85.
13. Rolling I, Lambjerg-Hansen H. Pulp condition of successfully formocresol-treated primary molars. Scand J Dent Res. 1978;86(4):267–72.
14. Ranly DM. Assessment of the systemic distribution and toxicity of formaldehyde following pulpotomy treatment: part one. J Dent Child. 1985;52:4331–4.
15. Myers D, Shoaf K, Dirksen T, Pashley DH, Whitford GM, Reynolds KE. Distribution of 14C-formaldehyde after pulpotomy with formocresol. J Am Dent Assoc. 1978;96:805–13.
16. Pashley E, Myers D, Pashley DH, Whitford G. Systemic distribution of 14C-formaldehyde from formocresol- treated pulpotomy sites. J Dent Res. 1980;59:602–8.
17. Milnes A. Is formocresol obsolete? a fresh look at the evidence concerning safety issues. Pediatr Dent. 2008;30:237–46.
18. Praveen K, Rashmi N, Vipin B, Pujan M. Pulpotomy medicaments: continued search for new alternatives- a review. Oral Health Dent Manag. 2014;13(4):883–90.
19. 's-Gravenmade EJ. Some biochemical considerations of fixation in endodontics. J Endod. 1973;1:233–7.
20. Kopel HM, Bernick S, Zachrisson E, De Romero SA. The effects of glutaraldehyde on primary pulp tissue following coronal amputation: an in vivo histological study. J Dent Child. 1980;47:425–30.
21. García-Godoy F. Clinical evaluation of glutaraldehyde pulpotomies in primary teeth. Acta Odontol Pediatr. 1984;4:41–4.
22. Fuks AB, Bimstein E, Klein H. Assessment of a 2 % buffered glutaraldehyde solution as a pulp dressing in pulpotomized human primary teeth. J Pedod. 1986;10:323–30.
23. Fuks AB, Bimstein E, Guelmann M, Klein H. Assessment of a 2 per cent buffered glutaraldehyde solution in pulpotomized primary teeth of school children. J Dent Child. 1990;57:371–5.
24. Davis MJ, Myers R, Switkes MD. Glutaraldeyde: an alternative to formocresol for vital pulp therapy. J Dent Child. 1982;49(3):176–80.
25. Lloyd MJ, Seale NS, Wilson CFG. The effects of various concentrations and lengths of application of glutaraldehyde on monkey pulp tissue. Pediatr Dent. 1988;10(2):115–20.
26. Fuks AB, Eidelman E, Cleaton-Jones P, Michaeli Y. Pulp response to ferric sulfate, diluted formocresol and IRM in pulpotomized primary baboon teeth. ASDC J Dent Child. 1997;64(4):254–9.
27. Fuks AB, Holan G, Davis JM, Eidelman E. Ferric sulfate versus dilute formocresol in pulpotomized primary molars: long-term follow up. Pediatr Dent. 1997;19:327–30.
28. Landau MJ, Johnson DC. Pulpal response to ferric sulfate in monkeys. J Dent Res. 1988;67:215 [Abstr #822].
29. Fei AL, Udin RB, Johnson R. A clinical study of ferric sulfate as a pulpotomy agent in primary teeth. Pediatr Dent. 1991;13(6):327–32.
30. Vargas K, Packham B. Radiographic success of ferric sulfate and formocresol pulpotomies and its relationship to early exfoliation. Pediatr Dent. 2005;27:233–337.
31. Vargas KG, Packham B, Lowman D. Preliminary evaluation of sodium hypochlorite for pulpotomies in primary molars. Pediatr Dent. 2006;28(6):511–7.
32. Rosenfeld EF, James GA, Burch BS. Vital pulp tissue response to sodium hypochlorite. J Endod. 1978;5:140–6.
33. Hafez AA, Kopel HM, Cox CF. Pulpotomy reconsidered: application of an adhesive system to pulpotomized permanent primate pulps. Quintessence Int. 2000;31:579–89.
34. Hafez AA, Cox CF, Tarim B, Otsuki M, Akimoto N. An in vivo evaluation of hemorrhage control using sodium hypochlorite and direct capping with a one or two component adhesive system in exposed nonhuman primate pulps. Quint Int. 2002;33(4):261–72.

35. Accorinte MLR, Loguercio AD, Reis A, Muench A, Araujo VC. Responses of human pulp capped with a bonding agent after bleeding control with hemostatic agents. Oper Dent. 2005;2:147–55.
36. Al-Mutairi MA, Bawazir OA. Sodium hypochlorite versus formocresol in primary molars pulpotomies: a randomized clinical trial. Eur J Ped Dent. 2013;14(1):33–6.
37. Ruby JD, Cox CF, Mitchell SC, Makhija S, Chompu-Inwai P, Jackson JA. Randomized study of sodium hypochlorite versus formocresol pulpotomy in primary molar teeth. Int J Ped Dent. 2013;23(2):145–52.
38. Shabzendedar M, Mazhari F, Alami M, Talebi M. Sodium hypochlorite vs formocresol as pulpotomy medicaments in primary molars: 1-year follow-up. Pediatr Dent. 2013;35(4): 329–32.
39. Zander HA. Reaction of the pulp calcium hydroxide. J Dent Res. 1939;18:373–9.
40. Magnusson B. Therapeutic pulpotomy in primary molars – Clinical and histological follow-up. I. Calcium hydroxide paste as wound dressing. Odontol Revy. 1970;21:415–31.
41. Schroder U. A 2-year follow-up of primary molars pulpotomized with a gentle technique and capped with calcium hydroxide. Scand J Dent Res. 1978;86:273–8.
42. Waterhouse PJ, Nunn JH, Whitworth JM. An investigation of the relative efficacy of Buckley's Formocresol and calcium hydroxide in primary molar vital pulp therapy. Br Dent J. 2000;188:32–6.
43. Ketley CE, Goodman JR. Formocresol toxicity: is there a suitable alternative for pulpotomy in primary molars? Int J Pediatr Dent. 1991;2:67–72.
44. Torabinejad M, Hong CU, McDonald F, Pitt Ford TR. Physical and chemical properties of a new root-end filling material. J Endod. 1995;21:349–53.
45. Sarkar NK, Caidedo R, Tirwik P, Moiseyeva R, Kawashima I. Physicochemical basis of the biologic properties of mineral trioxide aggregate. J Endod. 2005;31:97–100.
46. Torabinejad M, Hong CU, Pitt Ford TR, Kettering JD. Antibacterial effects of some root-end filling materials. J Endod. 1995;21:403–6.
47. Eidelman E, Holan G, Fuks AB. Mineral trioxide aggregate vs. formocresol in pulpotomized primary molars: a preliminary report. Pediatr Dent. 2001;23(1):15–8.
48. Parirokh M, Torabinejad M. Mineral trioxide aggregate: a comprehensive literature review-part III: clinical applications, drawbacks, and mechanism of action. Endod. 2011;36:400–13.
49. Smaïl-Faugeron V, Courson F, Durieux P, Muller-Bolla M, Glenny AM, Fron Chabouis H. Pulp treatment for extensive decay in primary teeth. Cochrane Database Syst Rev 2014;(8): 1–193.
50. International Agency for Research on Cancer. Press release no. 153. 15 Jun 2004. http://www.iarc.fr/pageroot/PRELEASES/pr153a.html.
51. Cvek M. A clinical report on partial pulpotomy and capping with calcium hydroxide in permanent incisors with complicated crown fracture. J Endod. 1978;4:232–7.
52. Cvek M, Cleaton-Jones PE, Austin JC, Andreasen JO. Pulp reactions to exposure after experimental crown fractures or grinding in adult monkeys. J Endod. 1982;8:391–7.
53. Holan G, McTique DJ. Introduction to dental trauma: managing traumatic injuries in the primary dentition. In: Casamassimo PS, Fields Jr HW, McTigue DJ, Nowak AJ, editors. Pediatric dentistry: infancy through adolescence. 5th ed. St. Louis: Elsevier Saunders; 2015. p. 213–30.
54. Fuks AB, Gavra S, Chosck A. Long-term followup of traumatized incisors treated by partial pulpotomy. Pediatr Dent. 1993;15:334–6.
55. Ram D, Holan G. Partial pulpotomy in a traumatized primary incisor with pulp exposure: case report. Pediatr Dent. 1994;16:44–8.
56. Petel R, Fuks A. Pink spot – A case report and literature review (in press) 2015.

Pulpectomy and Root Canal Treatment (RCT) in Primary Teeth: Techniques and Materials

6

Moti Moskovitz and Nili Tickotsky

Contents

M. Moskovitz, DMD, PhD (✉)
Department of Pediatric Dentistry, Hadassah Faculty of Dental Medicine,
The Hebrew University, 12272, Jerusalem 9112102, Israel
e-mail: motim@md.huji.ac.il

N. Tickotsky, DMD, MSc, MEd
The Goodman Faculty of Life Sciences, Nanotechnology Building, Bar Ilan University,
Ramat Gan 5290002, Israel
e-mail: nilitiko@gmail.com

A.B. Fuks, B. Peretz (eds.), *Pediatric Endodontics: Current Concepts in Pulp Therapy for Primary and Young Permanent Teeth*,
DOI 10.1007/978-3-319-27553-6_6

6.1 Introduction

When confronted with an infected and/or necrotic pulp in primary teeth, dentists have two options: the first is to extract the tooth and provide a space maintainer (when needed) to preserve space for the erupting permanent successor, and the other option includes removal of pulp remnants and root canal obturation followed by crown reconstruction. The lack of treatment is not an option as it can cause damage to the succedaneous tooth (e.g., enamel hypo-mineralization or hypoplasia) [1] and negatively impact the child's oral health-related quality of life (e.g., pain, eating preferences, quantity of food eaten, and sleep habits) [2].

As a rule, root canal treatment is indicated when the radicular pulp exhibits clinical signs of irreversible pulpitis or pulp necrosis, while the roots show minimal or no resorption [3], but we will also discuss cases in which a pulpectomy is recommended for teeth with a prognosis that is less than optimal.

Root canal treatment (RCT) is a technique-sensitive procedure, as instrumentation of the morphologically complicated canals of the primary molars encased in curved roots programmed for physiological resorption is quite challenging [4].

The following chapter will discuss the root canal treatment in primary teeth. Indications for treatment and root canal morphology as well as techniques and instruments used for canal cleansing and obturation will be reviewed. Special attention will be paid to possible adverse effects of RCT.

6.2 Morphological Considerations

Root canals of anterior primary teeth are relatively straight, have few irregularities, and are easily treated [5].

Primary maxillary molars may have two to four roots, with the three-rooted variant being the most common [4]. Fusion of the palatal and distobuccal roots occurs in approximately one-third of the primary maxillary first molars and occasionally in the primary maxillary second molars [5]

As shown in Fig. 6.1b, the primary maxillary first molars that have three roots (mesiobuccal (MB), distobuccal (DB), and palatal) have three canals. The palatal root is the longest and is curved, followed by the MB root. The DB root is the shortest and smallest in diameter [6, 7]. The physiologic root resorption causes the position of the apical foramen to change continually [5]. In addition, the presence of accessory canals makes biomechanical preparation difficult, and complete removal of necrotic pulp tissue is almost impossible (Fig. 6.1c).

Fig. 6.1 (**a**) Maxillary right first primary molar opened for RCT, showing the orifices of the three canals. (**b**) Maxillary right first primary molar, internal morphology (Courtesy of Prof. Eliezer Eidelman, Dr. Odont., M.S.D.). (**c**) Silicone models of maxillary first primary molars obtained after injection under pressure into the root canals and complete dissolution of the tooth material. Notice the intricate morphology of the root canal system

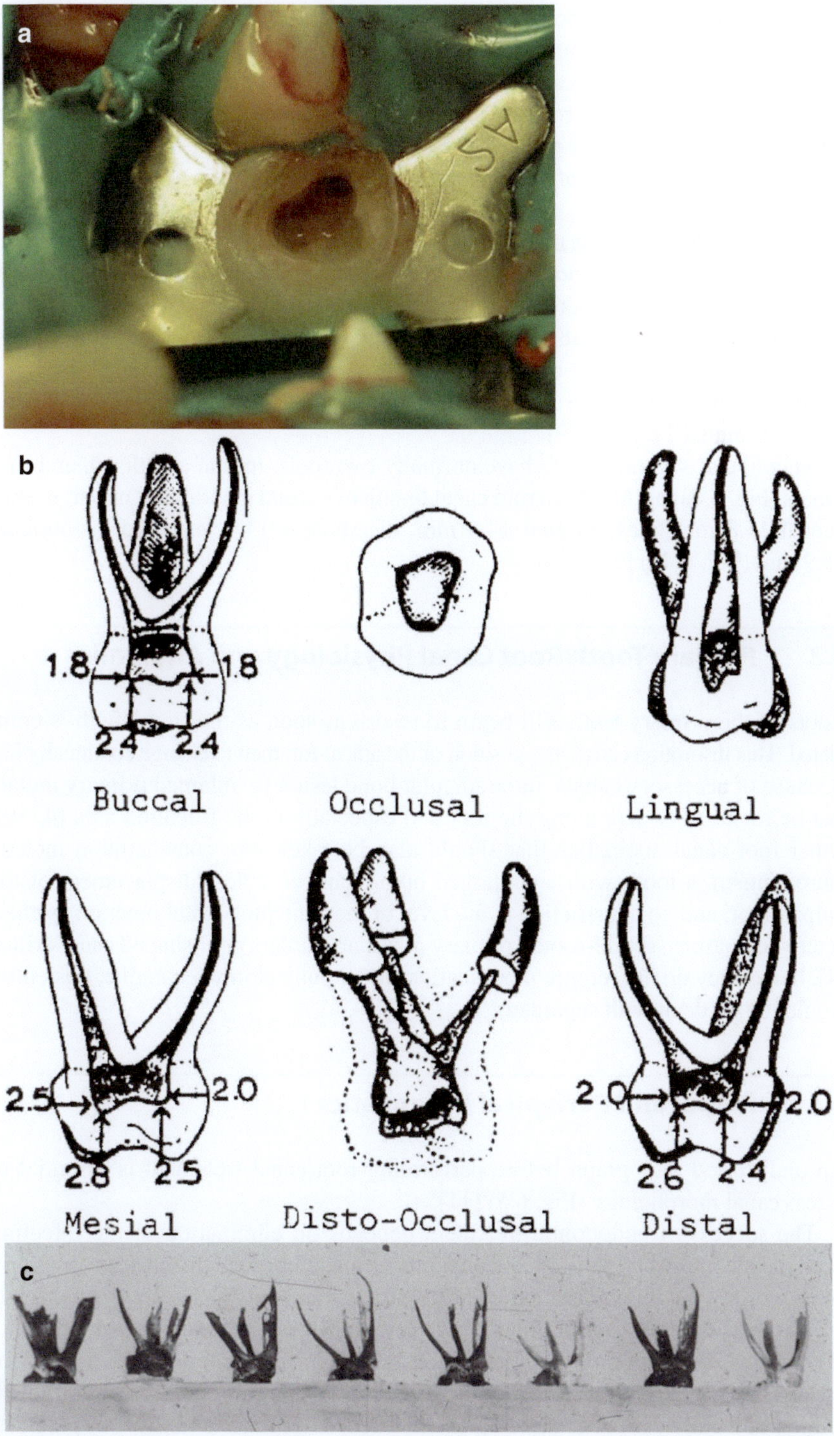
a
b
1.8
1.8
2.4
2.4
Buccal
Occlusal
Lingual
2.5
2.0
2.8
2.5
Mesial
Disto-Occlusal
2.0
2.0
2.6
2.4
Distal
c

Like the first primary molars, second primary maxillary molars (Fig. 6.2a) have three roots, and some exhibit fusion between the DB and palatal roots, with the palatal root being the longest, followed by the MBone. The DB root is the shortest and roundest of the three roots [6]. Second primary maxillary molars have either three canals (70 %) or four canals (30 %) (Fig. 6.2b) [8].

Mandibular primary molars can have one to three roots; the double-rooted variant is the most common.

Figures 6.3a, b illustrate mandibular first primary molars. Mandibular first molars have normally two roots; both are wider in the buccal-lingual dimension, narrower mesiodistally, and often grooved [6]. Mandibular first molars have either three canals (80 %) or four canals (20 %), the mesial roots usually have two root canals, and the distal root has one or two canals [4]. Mean root canal length of first mandibular molar: mesiobuccal 16.4 mm, mesiolingual 14.2 mm, distobuccal 13.1 mm, and distolingual 12.7 mm [9].

Mandibular second molars have normally two roots, mesial and distal, and four canals (Fig. 6.4a, b) [6]. Mean root canal length of second mandibular molar: mesiobuccal 15.8 mm, mesiolingual 14.4 mm, distobuccal 14.9 mm, and distolingual 14.9 mm (Fig. 6.4b) [9].

6.3 Primary Tooth Root Canal Physiology and Anomalies

Roots of the primary teeth will begin to resorb as soon as the root length is completed. This resorption causes the position of the apical foramen to change continually [5]. Because of accessory canals, interradicular bone lesion in inflamed primary molars can be found anywhere along the root and especially in the furcation area [4, 10]. Other root canal anomalies that should also be taken into consideration include taurodontism, a tooth with an enlarged pulp chamber, apical displacement of the pulpal floor, and no constriction at the level of the cementoenamel junction as characteristic features, single-rooted primary maxillary molars or C-shaped canal orifice [4], but as they do not require modification of the pulpectomy technique, this entity would not be dealt with separately.

6.4 Pulpal and Periapical Diagnostics

An undistorted radiograph before performing root canal treatment is essential to assess canal morphology (Fig. 6.5) [11].

The success of endodontic treatment depends on elimination of the infecting bacteria accomplished through adequate root canal debridement (instrumentation), antibacterial irrigations, and antibacterial filling materials [12]. Root canal treatment is considered successful if after a follow-up period the tooth (1) is not mobile; (2) remains in function without pain, discomfort, or infection until the permanent successor is ready to erupt; and (3) undergoes physiologic resorption [13]. Radiographically the tooth should present absence or reduction in size of preexisting pathologic radiolucent defects and no new lesions.

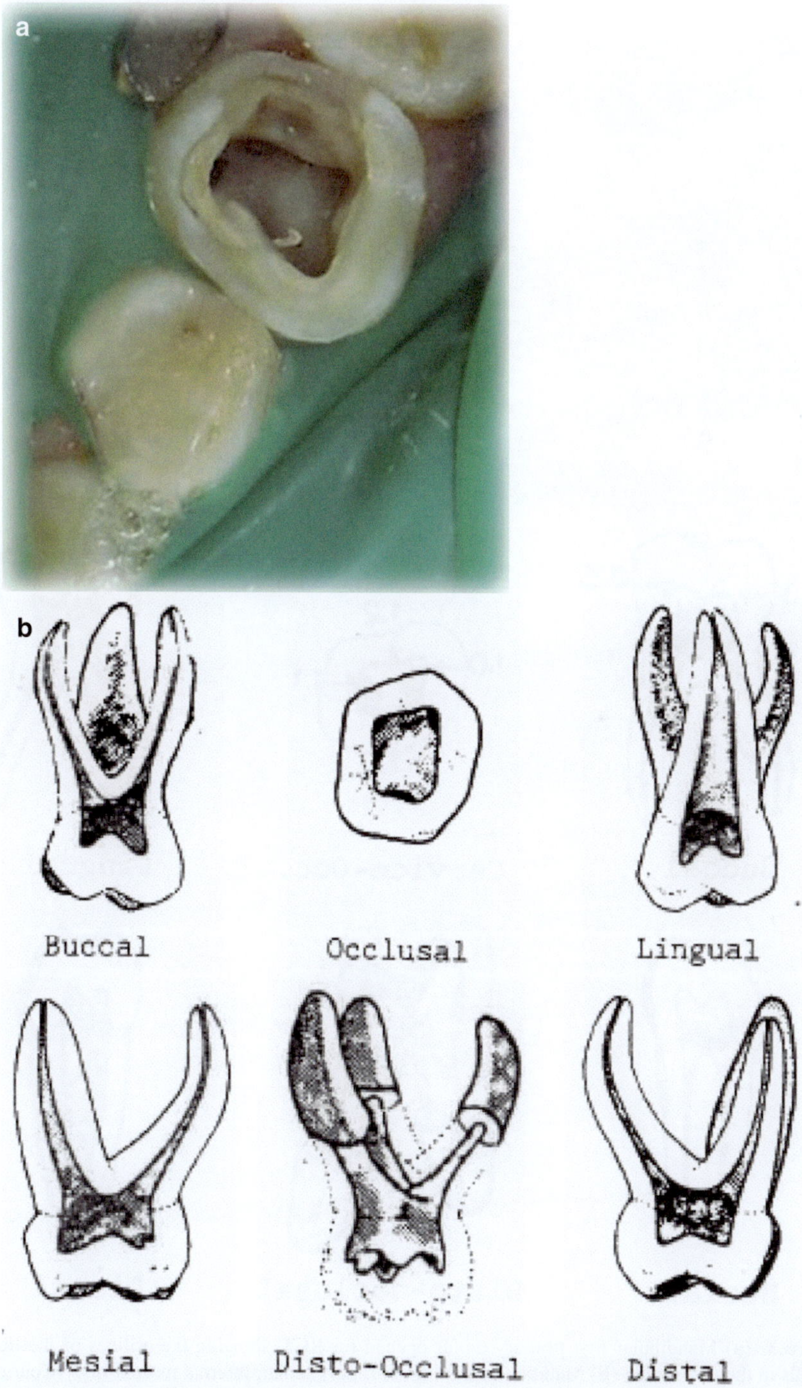

Fig. 6.2 (**a**) A second primary maxillary molar opened for RCT, showing the orifices of the three canals. (**b**) Maxillary right second primary molar, internal morphology (Courtesy of Prof. Eliezer Eidelman, Dr. Odont., M.S.D)

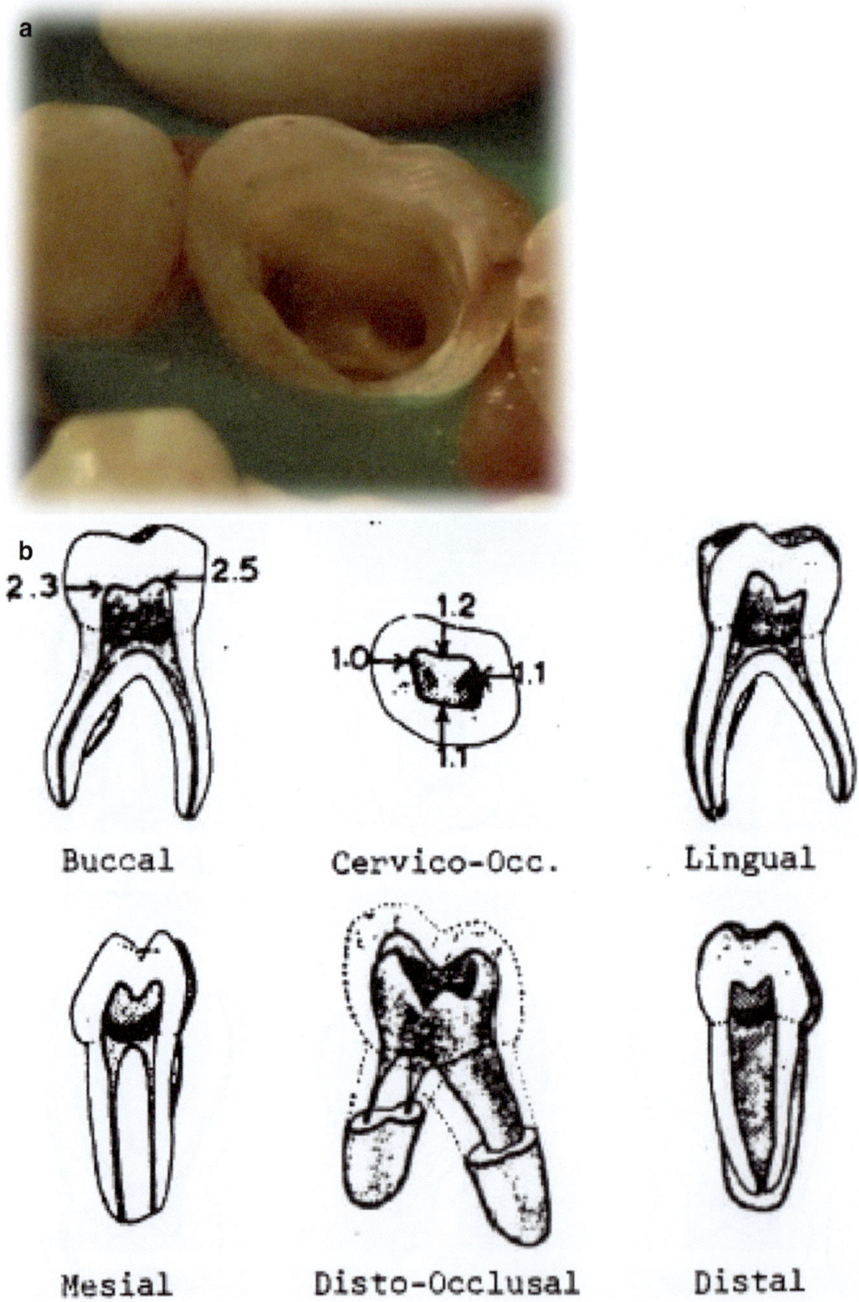

Fig. 6.3 (**a**) Mandibular first primary molar opened for RCT, showing the orifices of the three canals in the first molar. (**b**) Mandibular right first primary molar, internal morphology (Courtesy of Prof. Eliezer Eidelman, Dr. Odont., M.S.D)

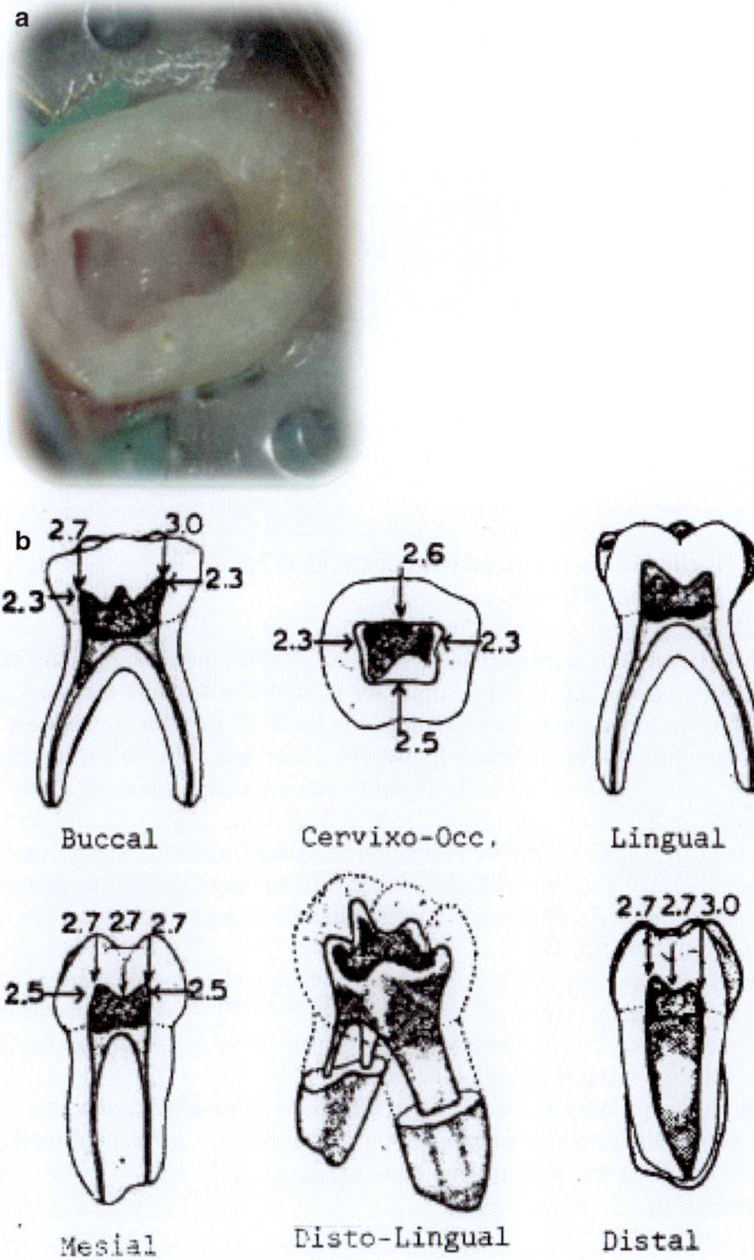

Fig. 6.4 (**a**) Mandibular second primary molar opened for RCT, showing the orifices of the three canals. (**b**) Mandibular second primary molar, internal morphology (Courtesy of Prof. Eliezer Eidelman, Dr. Odont., M.S.D)

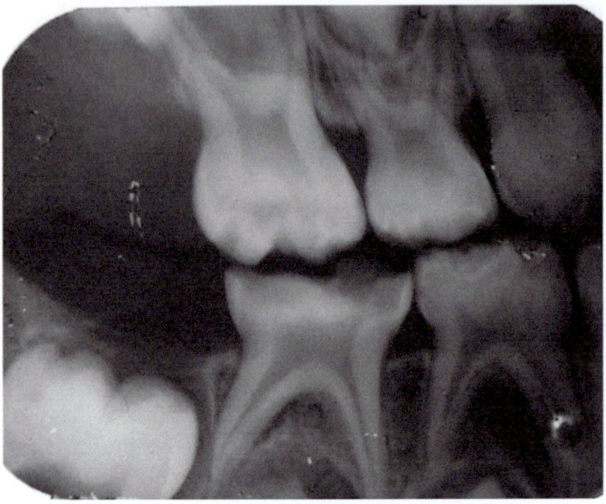

Fig. 6.5 The radiograph performed before root canal treatment (in this case, of the lower right second primary molar) should demonstrate the pulp chamber and the full length of the canals

6.5 Indications and Contraindications for RCT in Primary Teeth

Root canal treatment in primary teeth is indicated when the radicular pulp exhibits clinical signs of irreversible pulpitis or pulp necrosis, while the roots show minimal or no resorption. Contraindications for RCT in primary teeth are discussed lengthily in the literature [5, 13, 14]. Root canal treatment in primary molars is contraindicated in teeth: (1) with non-restorable crowns, (2) perforation to the pulpal floor, (3) serious reduction in bone support and/or extreme tooth mobility, (4) radiographic indication of extensive internal or external root resorption, (5) periradicular radiolucency involving the follicle of the permanent tooth, and (6) underlying dentigerous or follicular cysts and of medically compromised children [15, 16].

Lateral and accessory canals exist in most primary molars and are more prevalent in mandibular molars compared with maxillary ones [17]. Accessory canals in the furcation of primary molars can explain the frequent presence of radiolucency in the furcation area of necrotic of teeth [10, 18].

A RCT in a primary second molar with a poor prognosis is sometimes indicated, even if that tooth is maintained only until the first permanent molar has erupted, and then the primary molar is extracted and replaced with a space maintainer [19].

6.6 Root Canal Treatment (RCT) Techniques

RCT in primary teeth may be completed in one visit. Under local anesthesia and rubber dam isolation, caries is removed and access to the pulp chamber is gained.

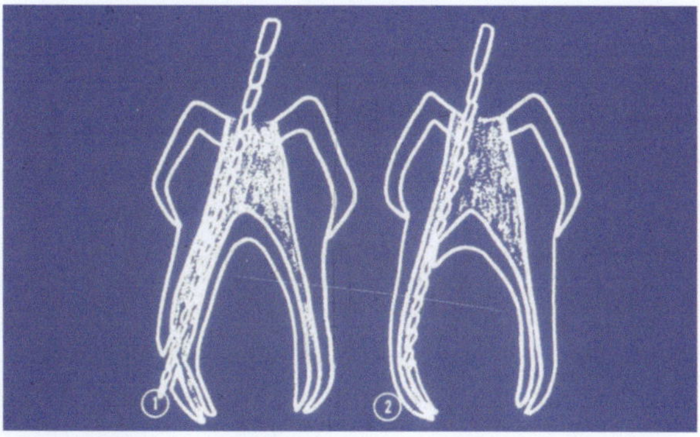

Fig. 6.6 Perforations on the convex (*1*) and concave (*2*) aspects of a root of a primary molar caused by injudicious use of root canal instruments

6.6.1 Access and Debridement

The inflamed or necrotic pulp is removed and access preparation is refined to make sure that entrance to all of the canals is possible and clearly visible.

Primary molar roots are usually curved to allow for the development of the succedaneous tooth. During instrumentation, these curves increase the chance of perforation of the apical portion of the root or the coronal one-third of the canal into the furcation [5]. After each canal orifice has been located, a properly sized barbed broach is selected. The broach is used gently to remove as much organic material as possible from each canal. Endodontic files are selected and adjusted to stop 1–2 mm short of the radiographic apex, with the preliminary working length estimated according to the preoperative radiograph. The instruments should be slightly bent to adjust to the curvature of the canals, thus preventing perforations on the outer and inner portions of the root (Fig. 6.6) [5].

Removal of organic debris is the main purpose of canal instrumentation. Mechanical removal of remnants from the canal is performed using a series of 21 mm long K-type endodontic files (Unitek Corp., Monrovia, CA) up to file No. 30 or 35 (Fig. 6.7). The initial working length is estimated with the x-ray. When the file is inserted into the canal, the apical stop is felt for with tactile sense and this measurement is then compared to the radiograph. Avoid unnecessary shaping of the canal since that can damage the tooth and lead to perforation in the furcation or the lateral walls.

6.6.2 Irrigation

Disinfection with irrigating solutions is an important step in assuring optimal bacterial decontamination of the canals. The root canals are irrigated with either 0.2 % up to 2 % chlorhexidine solution or with 1 % up to 5 % sodium hypochlorite (limited to one percent sodium hypochlorite according to the AAPD guidelines) (Fig. 6.8) [3, 4, 20–23].

The use of sodium hypochlorite in the primary dentition should be performed cautiously since it is a potent tissue irritant and must not be extruded beyond the apex [24–27] (Fig. 6.9).

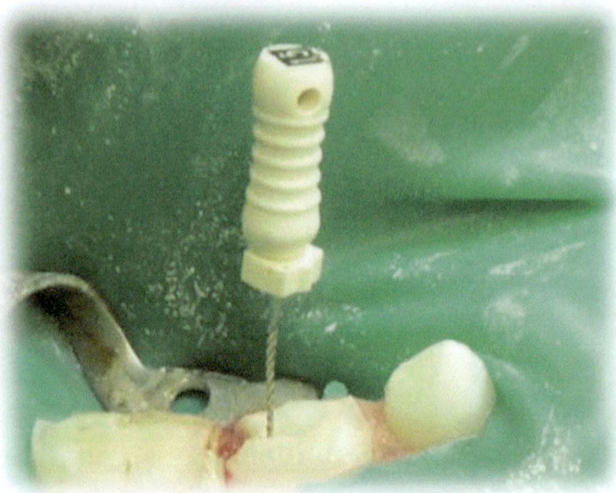

Fig. 6.7 Mechanical removal of remnants from the canal is performed using a series of 21 mm long K-type endodontic files (Unitek Corp., Monrovia, CA) up to file No. 30 or 35

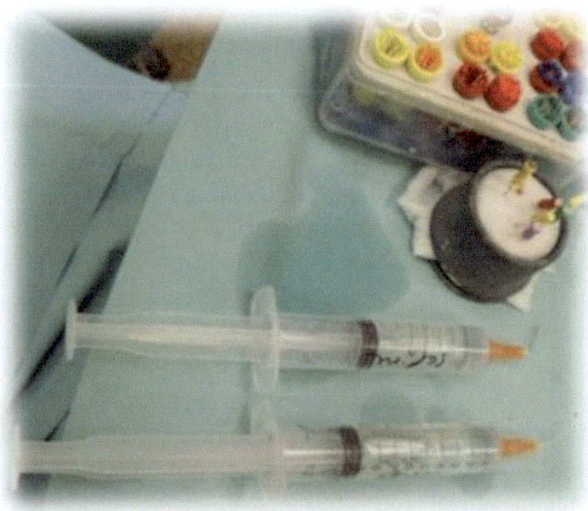

Fig. 6.8 The root canals are first irrigated with either 0.2 % up to 2 % chlorhexidine solution or with 1 % up to 5 % sodium hypochlorite and then with normal saline

Irrigation with normal saline before drying with appropriately sized sterile paper points (shown in Fig. 6.10) is also recommended. There is insufficient evidence supporting the outright superiority of any specific individual irrigation material or irrigating regime. Except anecdotal case reports, no evidence-based studies reported any adverse effects, and it is not clear if there were none or that they were just not reported, and thus the safety profile for each of the irrigating solutions remains unclear [28].

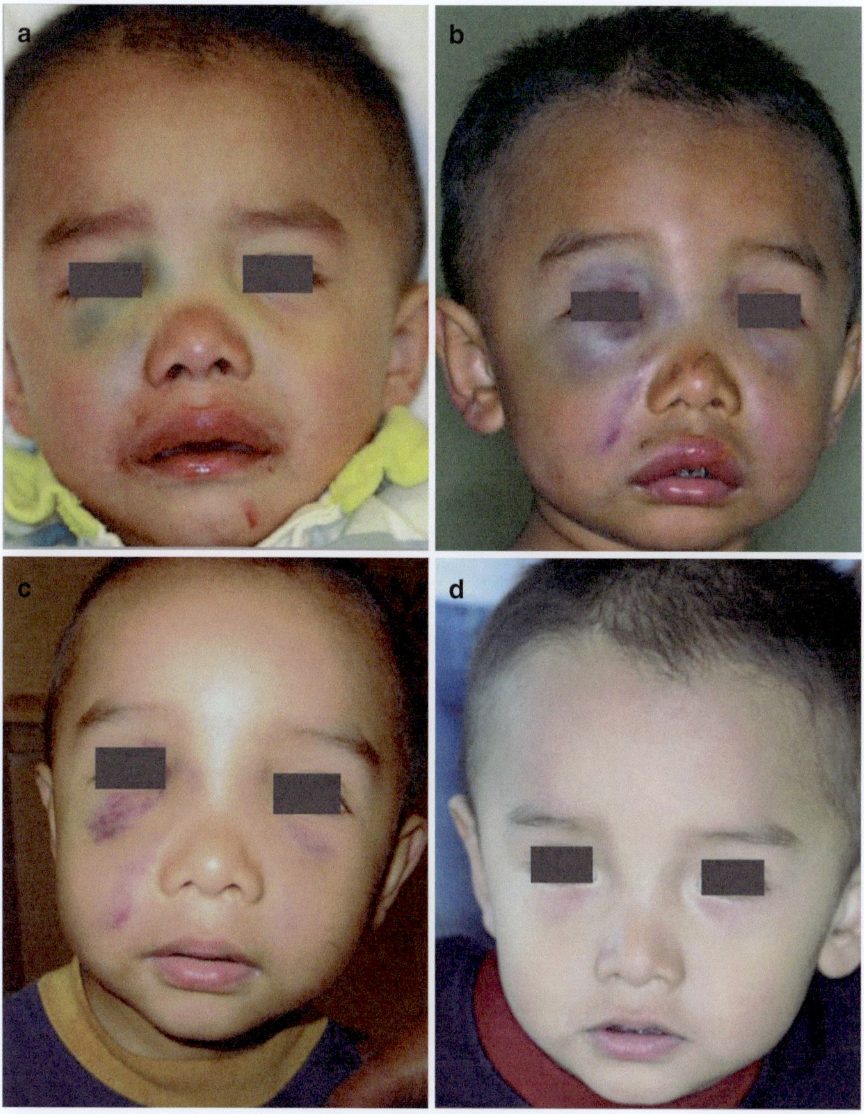

Fig. 6.9 Sodium hypochlorite accident in a pediatric patient. (**a**) Presentation in the postanesthesia care unit. (**b**) Presentation 1 day after the surgery. (**c**) Presentation 2 days after surgery. (**d**). Complete uneventful recovery 6 weeks after the surgery (Copyright © Klein and Kleier [26]. American Academy of Pediatric Dentistry and reproduced with their permission)

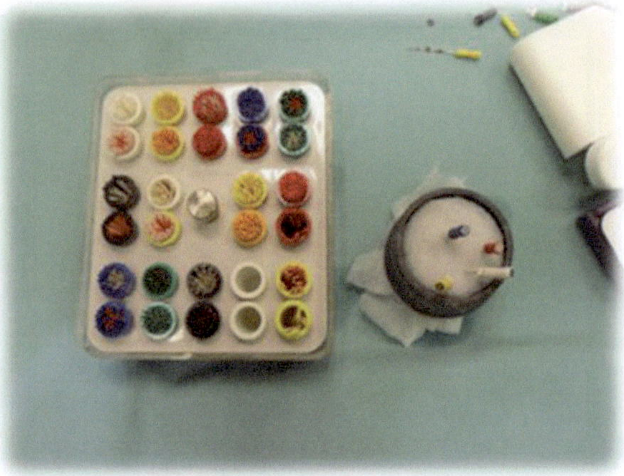

Fig. 6.10 Drying the canals should be performed with appropriately sized sterile paper points

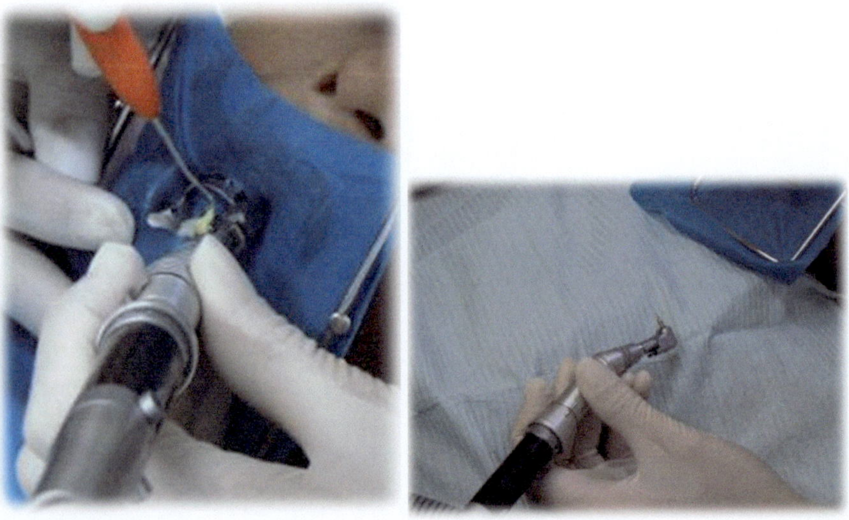

Fig. 6.11 Materials are inserted with a spiral lentulo mounted on a slow-speed engine

6.6.3 Filling the Canal(s)

The instruments employed to fill the canals depend mainly on the material used.

Thick paste such as ZOE is inserted and condensed with root canal pluggers, while thinner pastes like iodoform and calcium hydroxide-based materials are inserted with a spiral lentulo mounted on a slow-speed engine (Fig. 6.11: a spiral lentulo). Other materials are inserted with plastic syringes and tips provided by the manufacturer (Fig. 6.12: plastic syringe).

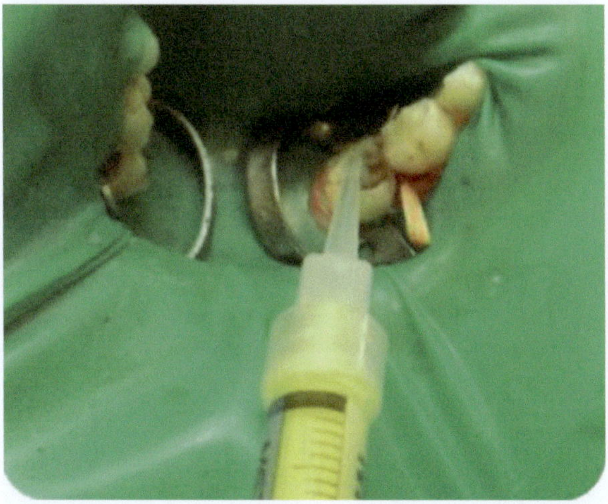

Fig. 6.12 Insertion of paste with a plastic syringe

6.7 Root Canal Filling Materials

The ideal root canal filling material should resorb at the same pace as the physiologic resorption of the roots, be nontoxic to the periapical tissues and to the permanent tooth germ, resorbs readily if forced beyond the apex and be antiseptic, easy to insert, nonshrinkable, and easily removed if necessary [19].

A number of root canal filling materials can be used for primary teeth, with no known ideal root canal filling material. Table 6.1 describes various popular root canal sealers for primary teeth. According to the literature, the most adequate material appears to be a calcium hydroxide-iodoform mixture [37]. Calcium hydroxide provides the high pH (>10) environment that, along with iodoform, has a high bacteriostatic effect [38].

The following paragraph describes several commonly used root canal filling materials. The characteristics of each material contribute its efficacy and biological behavior.

Zinc oxide-eugenol paste A thick mix of ZOE (Zinc Oxide BP, Eugenol BP, Associated Dental Products Ltd, Purton, England) without setting accelerators may be pushed into the root canals using a suitable root canal plugger. ZOE tends to resorb at a slower rate than the roots of the primary teeth [29–31], so placing it in the root canals can create a problem to the clinician: When extruded beyond the apices, the material sets into a hard cement that resists resorption (Fig. 6.13) [1, 39–42], it appeared in the tissue after loss of the pulpectomized tooth in 49.4 % of the cases [42], and it might remain in the alveolar bone for months or years (27.3 % of cases after a mean time of 40.2 months [42]). Remnants of ZOE may cause a mild foreign body reaction [43]. While in the USA, the use of ZOE without setting accelerators has been previously recommended [44]; currently the tendency is to use iodoform/calcium hydroxide filler [45].

Table 6.1 A description of various root sealers for primary teeth

Root filling material	Zinc oxide-eugenol	Calcium hydroxide with iodoform	Calcium hydroxide	Iodoform based	Zinc oxide and iodoform
Components		Vitapex (New Dental Chemical Products Co. Ltd., Tokyo, Japan)/ Diapex: 30 % calcium hydroxide, 40.4 % iodoform, and 22.4 % silicone oil.	Sealapex Calcicur	Metapex (Meta Biomed Co., Ltd. Cheongju City, Korea): calcium hydroxide with iodoform Kri paste(Pharmachemie AG, Switzerland): iodoform (80.8 %), camphor, parachlorophenol, menthol	Maisto's paste: zinc oxide and iodoform, with parachlorophenol camphor, lanolin, and thymol Endoflas (Sanlor & cfa. S. en C.S. from Columbia South America): tri-iodmethane and iodine dibutilorthocresol (40.6 %), zinc oxide (56.5 %), calcium hydroxide (1.07 %), and barium sulfate (1.63 %) with a liquid consisting of eugenol and paramonochlorophenol
Usage	Without setting accelerators may be pushed into the root canals using a suitable root canal plugger	Introduced into the root canal using disposable tips or a spiral lentulo mounted on a slow-speed handpiece	Introduced into the root canal using a spiral lentulo. Also available in automix syringes or application cannula	Sterile syringe with disposable plastic needles injects the paste into the canal	Introduced into the root canal using a spiral lentulo mounted on a slow-speed handpiece

Difficulties	Tends to resorb at a slower rate than the roots of the deciduous teeth [29–31]	Aqueous vehicles cause depletion of paste from root canals before the time of physiological tooth replacement [31][a] [a]Viscous vehicles promote lower solubility of the paste. Oily vehicles have lowest solubility and diffusion of calcium hydroxide pastes [32, 33]		Showed minimal antibacterial activity against most pure cultures [34] Overfilling and voids [35]	
Antibacterial activity	Strong antibacterial effectiveness [12, 36]	Showed no antibacterial activity against most pure cultures [36]		Kri paste showed stronger antibacterial effectiveness than did ZOE [36]	

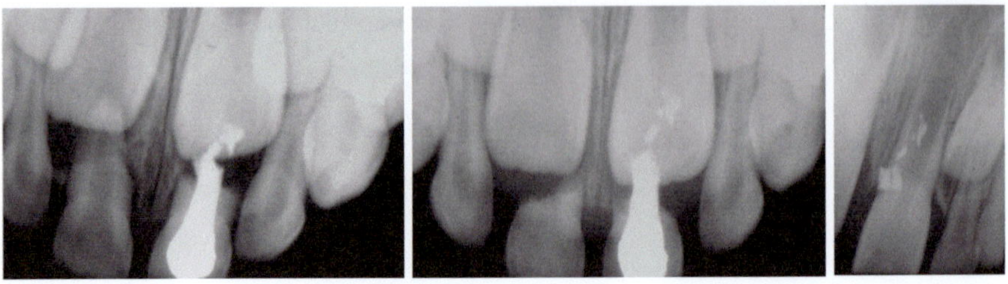

Fig. 6.13 ZOE extruded beyond the apices set into a hard cement that resists resorption (*left* and *center*). The remnants of the ZOE are still present after the eruption of the permanent central incisor

Calcium hydroxide pastes with iodoform The antimicrobial action of calcium hydroxide is associated with its ionic dissociation. The aqueous, viscous, or oily vehicle used in the formulation of the root canal filling paste impacts the speed of ionic dissociation. As aqueous vehicles favor a high degree of solubility, they will cause a depletion of the paste from the root canals *before* the time of physiological root resorption [31]. Viscous vehicles promote a lower solubility of the paste, and oily vehicles have the lowest solubility and diffusion of calcium hydroxide pastes showing better results [32, 33]. Iodoform-containing pastes such as Vitapex (pre-filled syringe with 0.5 g paste, Dia Dent Co., Tokyo, Japan) are introduced into the root canal using disposable tips or a spiral lentulo mounted on a slow-speed hand-piece, and the teeth are sealed with reinforced zinc oxide-eugenol (IRM – L.D. Caulk, Dentsply Milford, DE). Vitapex is a combination of 30 % calcium hydroxide, 40.4 % iodoform, and 22.4 % silicone oil. It is radiopaque, premixed, easy to use (plastic syringe tip) (Fig. 6.12) and to remove and absorbed if inadvertently extruded past the apex [38]. In primary teeth with irreversible pulpal changes, ZOE pulpectomies yielded similar outcomes as Vitapex and more favorable than Sealapex, a calcium hydroxide cement (SybronEndo, Orange, CA), although there was no agreement with regard to filling materials' resorption [46]. Vitapex is sold in North America as Diapex (DiaDent Group International, Burnaby, BC, Canada). When extruded into furcal or apical areas, it can either diffuse or be resorbed in 1 or 2 weeks. Bone regeneration has been clinically and histologically documented [47]. Tchaou et al. employed pure cultures of bacteria that have been reported to inhabit non-vital root canals of primary teeth and found that Vitapex did not inhibit the growth of *S. mutans*, *S. aureus*, or *L. casei* and showed no antibacterial activity against most pure cultures [36].

Iodoform-based pastes In vitro studies found that Metapex demonstrated minimal inhibition of 23 strains of bacteria isolated from infected root canals of primary molars and three nonstandard bacterial strains using agar diffusion assay [34] compared with zinc-oxide eugenol paste and materials containing zinc oxide [48].

Maisto's paste, introduced in 1967, includes both zinc oxide and iodoform, with parachlorophenol camphor, lanolin, and thymol. The presence of zinc oxide slows it resorption, and it was reported to have significantly higher success rates (100 %) compared to ZOE alone [38, 49, 50].

KRI paste (Pharmachemie, Zurich) is a mixture of iodoform (80.8 %), camphor, parachlorophenol, and menthol [38, 51, 52]. KRI paste showed stronger antibacterial effectiveness than did ZOE against pure cultures of obligate anaerobes with *Bacteroides* (currently *Porphyromonas Prevotella)* species and anaerobic streptococci isolated from non-vital root canals of primary teeth [36].

6.8 Supplementary Methods

Dental operating microscopes, electronic apex locators, rotary nickel-titanium files and irrigation techniques are at the front of endodontic armamentarium today [4, 13, 53–64].

The use of dental operating microscope [4] is not essential when treating primary teeth. Preparation of root canals in primary teeth (contrary to permanent teeth) is based on chemical means rather than on mechanical debridement [13].

When considering the use of electronic apex locators, only few studies exist and most of them are either in vitro [53, 65] or studies performed under general anesthesia [54, 55, 66–68]. Those studies recommend further evaluation of the application of apex locators in primary teeth, but as of now it is not yet an established procedure.

As for rotary instrumentation techniques in primary molars, in vitro studies found equal cleaning capacity but reduction of instrumentation time by the rotary technique [56–60]. The use of the rotary technique reduced the time of instrumentation and obturation to 63 and 68 %, respectively, and also improved the quality of the root canal filling [56, 61, 63]. The reduction of RCT procedure time is a relevant clinical factor in the treatment of children, but, due to lack of in vivo appropriate studies, it is not yet possible to recommend the use of rotatory filing technique as a standard procedure.

Er,Cr:YSGG laser provided similar cleanliness as rotary instrumentation technique and was superior to manual instrumentation. The laser technique required less time for completion of the cleaning and shaping procedures when compared with both rotary or hand instrumentation [64]. Here too, due to the limited clinical studies and the lack of adequate follow-up, this technique cannot be yet recommended for common practice, and so manual instrumentation is still the preferred debridement method for root canals in US dental schools and practiced by Diplomats of the American Board of Pediatric Dentistry in the USA [45].

6.9 Evaluation of RCT

RCT is considered successful if clinically pretreatment clinical signs and symptoms resolve within a few weeks and the tooth is painless, presenting healthy surrounding soft tissues and no increased mobility. The treatment should permit resorption of the roots of the primary tooth and filling material and allow normal eruption of the succedaneous tooth.

Radiographic lesions present preoperatively should resolve within 6 months, as evidenced by bone deposition and a decrease or disappearance or at least no change in pretreatment radiolucent areas. No pathologic root resorption, furcation/apical radiolucency [31, 50], or new lesion should appear after treatment.

Radiographically, success is defined either as when the radiolucency observed at the baseline did not increase [69] or is decreased in size [30, 70, 71] or when there is no radiolucency in the furcal or periradicular areas In all trials, success rates were equal to or above 78 %.

Treatment is considered a failure when preexisting radiolucent defects have grown in size or new defects appeared.

Success rate of root canal treatments in primary teeth has been discussed in the literature. Success rates were around 53 % in an early study [72] that used a different technique than the average pulpectomy that is performed today. Later studies have reported success rates of 95 and 99 % [5]. More recent studies achieved a success rate of 82 to 90 % for primary molar RCT with a ZOE filling material [73, 74]. The success rate of RCT in the anterior teeth varied from 76 to 82.8 % [1, 30, 75–78]. When using Kri Paste, the rate of successful treatments with no clinical or radiographic signs or symptoms was from over 80 % up to as high as 95.6 % [16, 40, 41, 51, 79–81].

In a review article by Barcelos et al., the overall success of pulpectomy was 80.0 % for Calcicur (a calcium hydroxide paste), 60.0 % for Sealapex and varied from 85.0 to 100.0 % for ZOE and from 89.0 to 100.0 % for Vitapex. Calcicur presented a significantly lower success rate when compared to ZOE and Vitapex. These pastes lead to overfilled canals, and particles of extruded ZOE were still evident even after the evaluation period. Resorption of Vitapex, Calcicur, and Sealapex within the root canal was also reported [46].

Cochrane review of clinical and radiographic follow-up up to 24 month of 13 comparisons between different medicaments for pulpectomy in primary teeth (eight trials) did not find sufficient evidence to establish superiority of one medicament over the other with regard to clinical failure [82].

Endoflas and zinc oxide-eugenol showed 93.3 % success, whereas a higher percentage of success was observed with Metapex (100 %) [35]. The success rates with ZOE varied between 65 and 100 % with an average of 83 % [19, 30, 31, 33, 50, 51, 69–71, 83]. For success rates of RCT with various sealers, see Table 6.2.

Regarding RCT procedure, as of 1997, 98 % of US dental schools were teaching hand instrumentation of canals, with the majority of schools not recommending any enlargement of the canal. The most commonly recommended irrigators were sodium hypochlorite, sterile water or saline, and local anesthetic. Ninety percent of schools recommended ZOE as the preferred filling for root canals [44].

6.9.1 Postoperative Radiographic Evaluation

A postoperative periapical radiograph is performed to determine the adequacy of the root canal filling and to determine the extent of root canal filling material in the

Table 6.2 Success rates of RCT with various sealers

Root filling material	Zinc oxide-eugenol	Calcium hydroxide with iodoform	Calcium hydroxide	Iodoform based	Zinc oxide and iodoform
Publications	Fuks (2012), Holan (1993), Mani (2000), Mortazavi (2004), Ozalp (2005), Damle (2005), Reddy (1996), Trairatvorakul (2008), Barja-Fidalgo (2011), Rewal (2014)	Ramar (2010), Subramaniam (2011), Chen (2012)	Barcelos (2011)	Ramar (2010), Subramaniam (2011), Chen (2012)	Mass (1989), Reddy (1996), Chen (2012), Moskovitz (2005)
Success rates	65–100 %, 83 % average	Vitapex: 90.5–100 %	60 %	Metapex: 90.5–100 % KRI paste: 84 %	Maisto's paste: 100 % Endoflas: 93.3 %

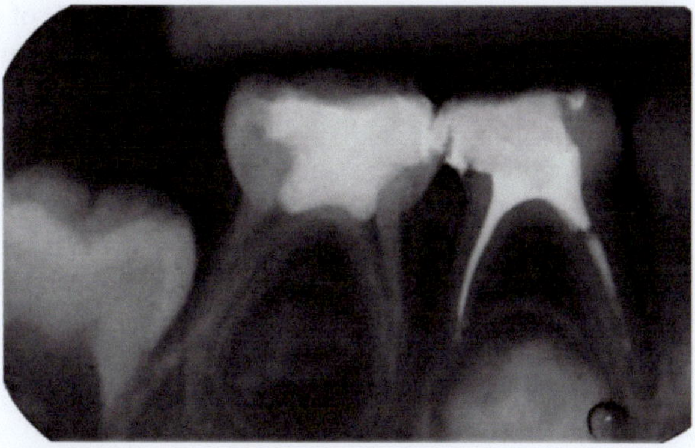

Fig. 6.14 A postoperative periapical radiograph is performed to determine the adequacy of the root canal filling and to determine the extent of root canal filling material in the canals. The filling in the distal canal is "flush," while the mesial is slightly underfilled

canals (Fig. 6.14). "Flush" is the ideal state, in which the filling material reaches the radiographic apex of the roots without being extruded beyond the apex, "under fill" is when the filling material does not reach the apex, and "overfill" when the filling material extends beyond the apex (Fig. 6.15).

The tooth is then restored either at the same appointment or as soon as possible. If restoration is postponed and not performed at the same appointment and the tooth is asymptomatic, the root-treated primary molars are restored in the following appointment with a leakage-free restoration, preferably a stainless steel crown (amalgam, composite, or reinforced glass ionomer restorations may apply provided they are microleakage-free). The crown can be restored with one of the abovementioned restoration materials if sufficient crown structure is left to retain the restoration. Otherwise, a stainless-steel crown is indicated.

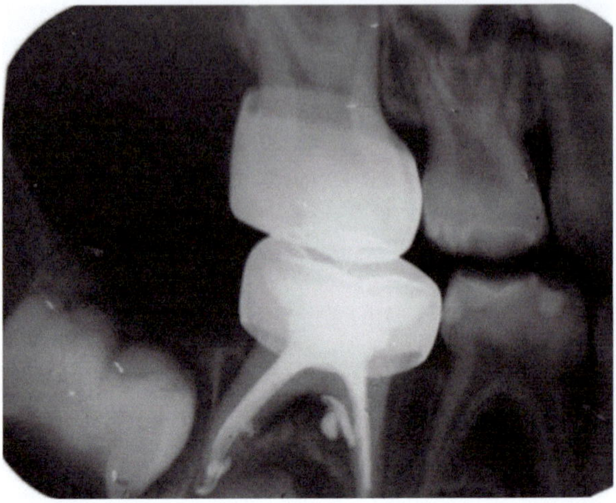

Fig. 6.15 In an overfilled root, the filling material extends beyond the apex

6.9.2 Antibiotics in Endodontics

The vast majority of teeth with symptomatic apical periodontitis or an acute apical abscess can be effectively managed without the use of antibiotics. The first line of treatment should be removal of the source of inflammation or infection by local, operative measures [84]. Penicillin is ineffective for pain relief [85]. Antibiotics are not recommended for healthy patients with symptomatic pulpitis, symptomatic apical periodontitis, a draining sinus tract, a localized swelling of endodontic origin, or following endodontic surgery [86]. There is concern that dentists who continue to prescribe unnecessary antibiotics could contribute to the development of antibiotic-resistant bacteria [84, 87]. Systemic antibiotics are currently only recommended for situations where there is evidence of spreading infection (cellulitis, lymph node involvement, diffuse swelling) or systemic involvement (fever, malaise) [86].

6.9.3 Degree of Root Resorption After Root Canal Treatments

Root canal treatment using iodoform-containing root canal filling material was found to accelerate root resorption [88]. This is in accordance with the findings that local factors like decay, pulp necrosis, and pulpotomy hastened the rate of root resorption of the primary molars [89].

6.10 Adverse Effects of Root Canal Treatments in Primary Teeth

The influences of root canal treatments in primary teeth on the development of the permanent tooth bud and the eruption of the permanent tooth have hardly been studied. Overfilling may cause a mild foreign body reaction, and it has also been associated with an increased failure rate when compared to underfilling or flush finishing [19, 51].

Studies have shown that remnants of ZOE may be found in the alveolar bone in 50 % and up to 70 % of the exfoliated primary teeth, and this material was still retained in more than a quarter of the patients after three years [16, 42, 79]. Figure 6.13 demonstrates a case of a ZOE-overfilled primary central incisor whose remnants remained in the tissue even after the eruption of the succedaneous permanent incisor.

According to Coll and Sadrian, RCT correctly done do not cause adverse effects on the succedaneous teeth, but have a 20 % chance of altering the path of permanent tooth eruption when using ZOE filling material [1]. Incorrectly performed root canal treatment may cause arrest of eruption of the succedaneous teeth [90]. Ectopic eruption of permanent incisors following ZOE pulpectomy of their primary predecessors was also described by Tannure et al. [91].

It could be hypothesized that ectopic eruption of a permanent incisor might not be caused by a RCT on the primary incisor but due to severe trauma to the primary incisor affecting and/or dislodging the developing permanent bud.

Studies have shown either no or low incidence of enamel hypoplasia in succedaneous teeth when the primary teeth have been treated with pulpectomy [1, 16].

Failure of root canal treatment occurred in 3.3 % of the primary molars that presented with a new radiolucent lesion or enlargement of existing periapical radiolucency after being treated with zinc oxide and iodoform paste. When a periradicular radiolucent lesion is present before the RCT, the likelihood of failure (e.g., increase in size of the lesion) is higher than in the absence of such a defect before the treatment. No association was found between RCT in primary molars and the appearance of enamel defects or ectopic eruption of the following premolars [92].

Previous studies raised the possibility of radicular cysts developing in concurrence with low-grade irritation to the dental sac of a permanent successor by root canal filling material leaking from resorbed primary apices [92, 93]. In those studies, enlargement of the dental sac in association with a root-treated primary tooth occurred in 3.3 % of the followed cases, but the development of a true radicular or dentigerous cysts was a rare occasion. Despite the low occurrence, dentists should be aware of this phenomenon and radiographically monitor root canal treated teeth until shedding (Fig. 6.16).

Most radicular cysts in the primary dentition do not demonstrate clinical signs, but if the cyst attains a certain size, displacement of the developing tooth bud might occur [1, 14, 94, 95], accompanied by expansion of the buccal cortical plate (Fig. 6.17) [94, 95].

6.10.1 RCT in Canines and Incisors

Iodoform pastes have better resorbability and disinfectant properties than ZOE, but commonly produce a dark-brown discoloration of the tooth crowns compromising the esthetics [30, 33, 96].

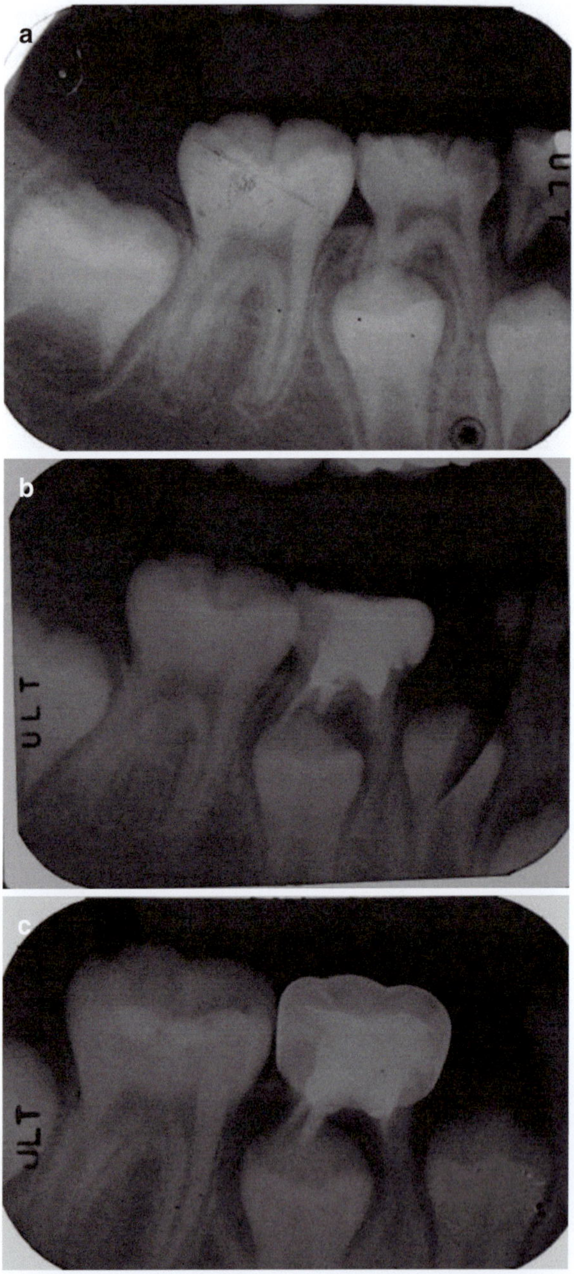

Fig. 6.16 Root canal treatment using Endoflas, performed in a primary right second mandibular molar. Figures (**a**, **b**) are pre- and postoperative radiographs. Radiograph (**c**) demonstrates enlargement of the dental sac of the mandibular right second premolar 3 months later

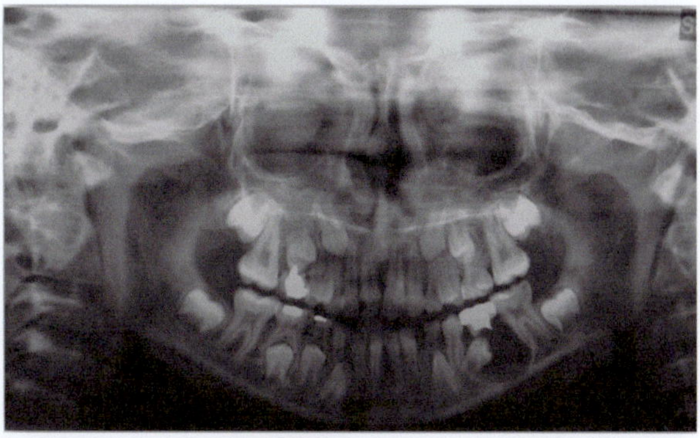

Fig. 6.17 A radicular cyst associated with a lower second primary molar with a root canal treatment. The tooth germ is deflected mesially. The large cystic lesion may endanger the lower border of the mandible (Courtesy of Emanuel Twito, DMD)

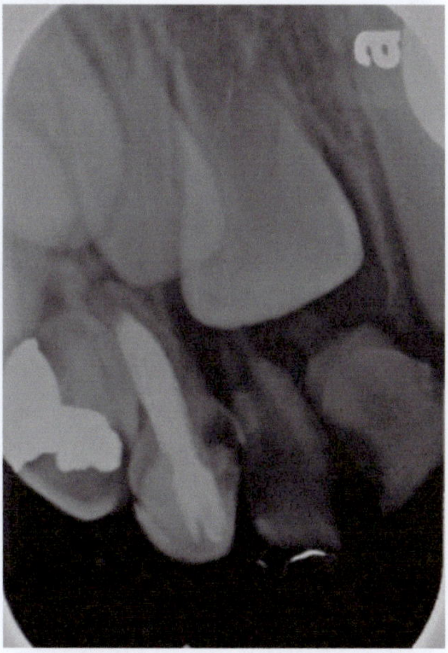

Fig. 6.18 Primary right canine with a classic SURTEX® Dentatus prefabricated metal post (Courtesy of Maya Dotan, DMD)

6.10.2 Metal Post

Figure 6.18 illustrates a primary upper right canine with a classic SURTEX® Dentatus prefabricated metal post. This procedure is not acceptable in primary teeth as the roots are predestined to resorb and the metal post may injure the permanent tooth bud. Furthermore the post and core are not leakage-free and as demonstrated in this case. The root canal filling material is washed away from the canal exposing it to reinfection. In case of unrestorable teeth, the preferred option is extraction.

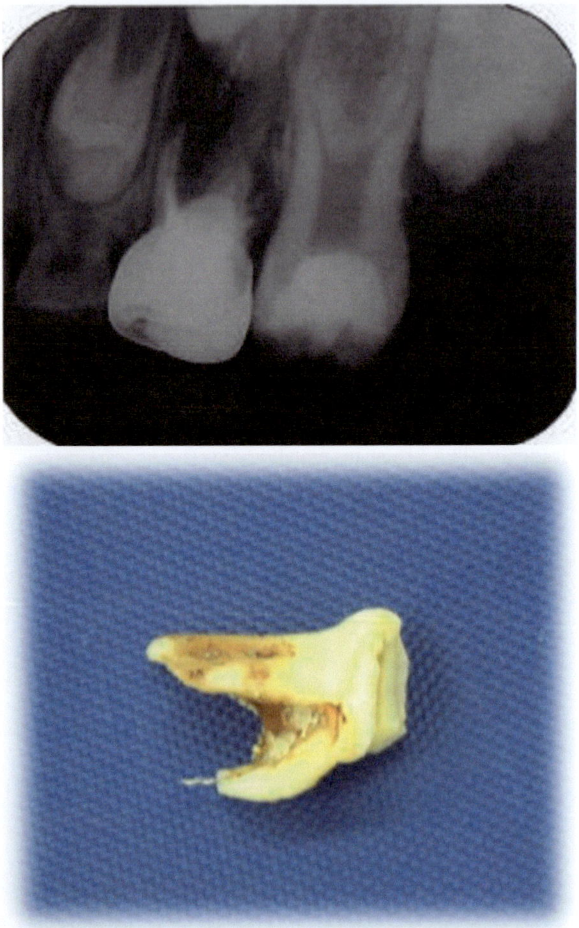

Fig. 6.19 (**a**) Radiographic view of a broken lentulo spiral filler in a canal post RCT. (**b**) The tooth was extracted. The lentulo spiral filler is bulging from the apex

6.10.3 Lentulo Spiral Fillers

Lentulo spiral fillers are dental instruments with constantly spaced spirals used to distribute sealer or cement in root canals. Care must be taken to avoid the possibility of the spiral breaking inside the root canal. Clinicians should always perform correct use of the instrument especially in primary teeth with tortuous root canals and dispose of old instruments. In case of a broken instrument in the canal, one should consider extracting the tooth or performing a close follow-up and extracting the tooth as soon as the tooth bud is approaching the edge of the lentulo in the resorbing root (Fig. 6.19).

6.10.4 Turner Tooth

An enamel defect in the permanent teeth caused by periapical inflammatory infection in the overlying primary tooth is referred to as Turner's tooth. Turner's hypoplasia is the result of disruption in the process of enamel matrix formation, which in

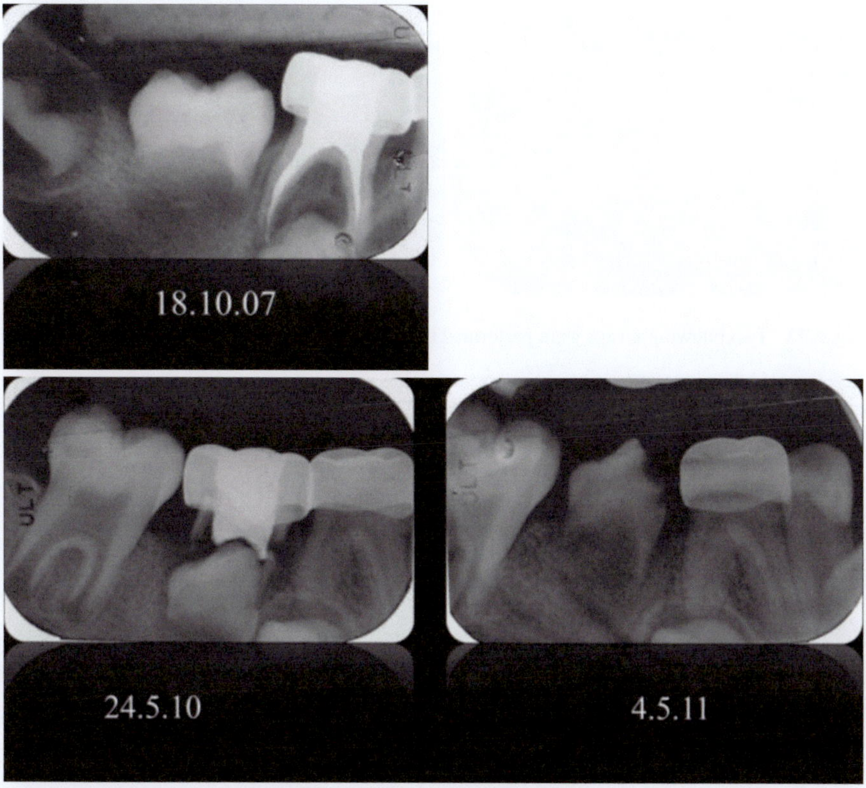

Fig. 6.20 Although rare, hypoplasia in the permanent successor as a sequela to a RCT in a primary tooth may occur even after a successful RCT (Courtesy of Gal Wallenstein, DMD)

turn causes both quality and thickness of enamel to be defective (See Chap. 2). Turner's hypoplasias in permanent teeth that resulted from periapical lesions in non-vital primary teeth have been reported [97].

Although rare, hypoplasia in the permanent successor as a sequela to a RCT in a primary tooth may occur even after a successful RCT. Those incidences emphasize the crucial need for periodical follow-up visits to evaluate the treated primary tooth (Fig. 6.20).

6.11 Case: Root Canal Treatment in a Primary Molar

A healthy 5-year-old Caucasian boy presented at the clinic. Patient appeared apprehensive and uncooperative, objecting dental examination. Father stated that the child "had severe pain awaking him from sleep a few weeks ago." Intraoral examination revealed soft tissue swelling and redness around the lower right primary first molar.

Two bitewing x-rays were performed (periapical x-rays of the lower right second primary molar was not taken) (Fig. 6.21). Based on the history of pain, the clinical examination, and radiographic findings, the most probable diagnosis was exacerbation of chronic dentoalveolar abscess in the lower right first primary molar.

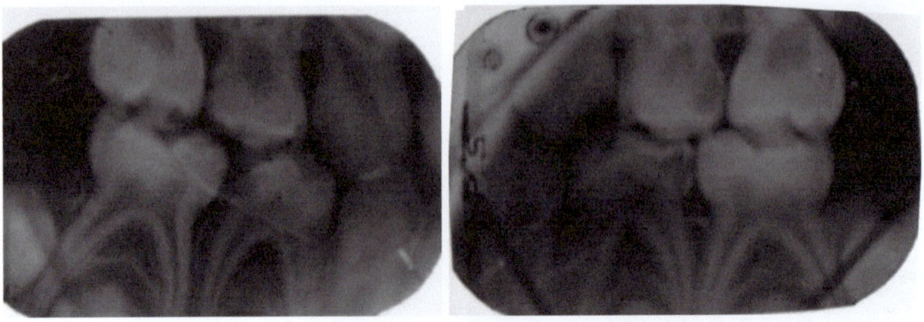

Fig. 6.21 Two bitewing x-rays were performed the first time the child presented, 30.8.12

Fig. 6.22 RCT was performed as an emergency treatment in the lower right mandibular first primary molar, 30.8.12

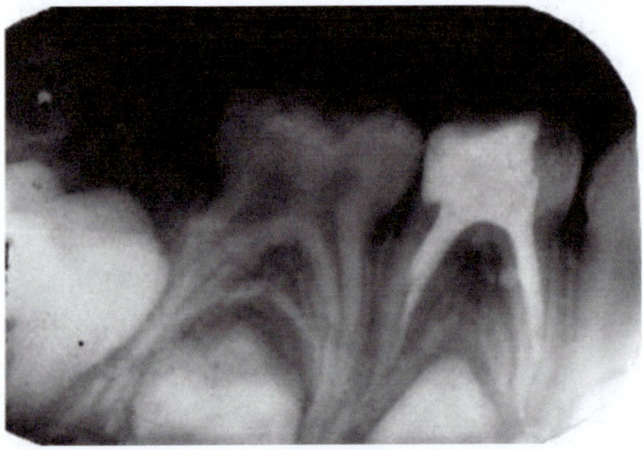

Fig. 6.23 Post-op x-ray of RCT in the lower left mandibular first primary molar, 23.5.13

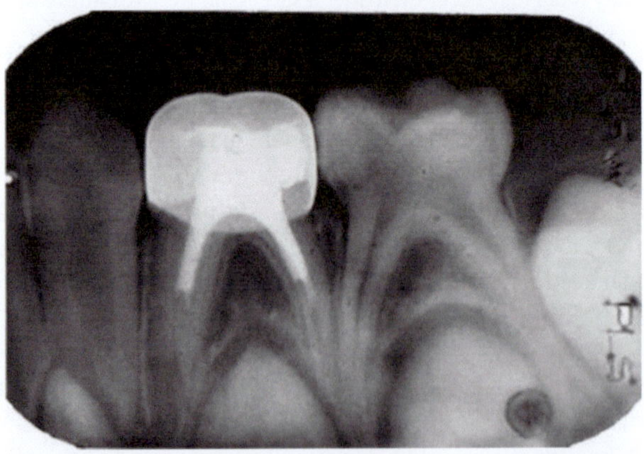

On the same appointment, using conscious sedation, RCT was performed as an emergency treatment in the lower right mandibular first primary molar (Fig. 6.22). Due to parents delaying the next appointment, another emergency treatment using conscious sedation was performed, this time a RCT in the lower left mandibular first primary molar (Fig. 6.23). Comprehensive treatment of other carious lesions was accomplished using inhaled sedation.

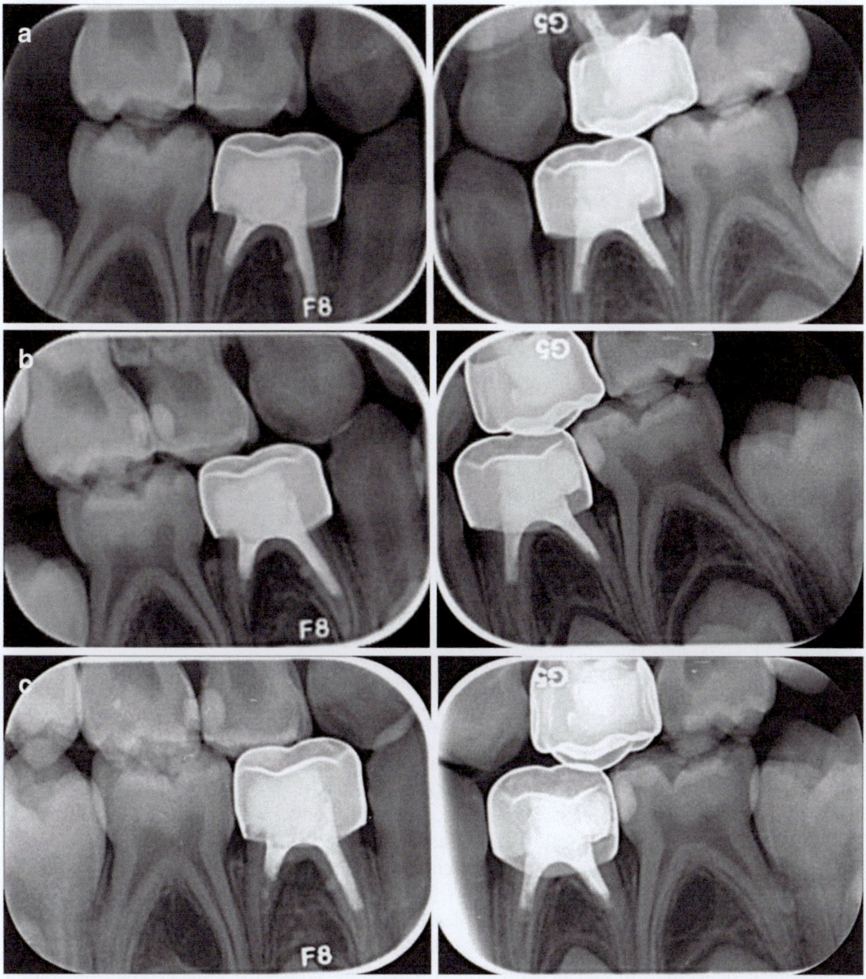

Fig. 6.24 Recall appointments demonstrated new carious lesions that needed treatment, but both (lower first mandibular teeth) RCT teeth appeared to have no clinical or radiographic pathologies. (**a**) First recall appointment after 15 month, (**b**) Second recall appointment 23 months after treatment and (**c**) Third recall appointment 2 years and 9 months after the RCT treatment.

During the next 2 years and 9 month, recall appointments demonstrated new carious lesions that needed treatment, but both (lower first mandibular teeth) RCT teeth appeared to have no clinical or radiographic pathologies (Fig. 6.24).

References

1. Coll JA, Sadrian R. Predicting pulpectomy success and its relationship to exfoliation and succedaneous dentition. Pediatr Dent. 1996;18(1):57–63.
2. Low W, Tan S, Schwartz S. The effect of severe caries on the quality of life in young children. Pediatr Dent. 1999;21(6):325–6.

3. American Academy of Pediatric Dentistry: guideline on pulp therapy for primary and young permanent teeth. Revised 1998, 2001, 2004, 2009, 2014. Pediatr Dent. 242–50.
4. Ahmed HMA. Anatomical challenges, electronic working length determination and current developments in root canal preparation of primary molar teeth. Int Endod J. 2013;46(11):1011–22.
5. Goerig AC, Camp JH. Root canal treatment in primary teeth: a review. Pediatr Dent. 1983;5(1):33–7.
6. Cleghorn BM, Boorberg NB, Christie WH. Primary human teeth and their root canal systems. Endod Top. 2010;23(1):6–33.
7. Zoremchhingi, Joseph T, Varma B, Mungara J. A study of root canal morphology of human primary molars using computerised tomography: an in vitro study. J Indian Soc Pedod Prev Dent. 2005;23(1):7–12.
8. Aminabadi NA, Farahani RMZ, Gajan EB. Study of root canal accessibility in human primary molars. J Oral Sci. 2008;50(1):69–74.
9. Salama FS, Anderson RW, McKnight-Hanes C, Barenie JT, Myers DR. Anatomy of primary incisor and molar root canals. Pediatr Dent. 1992;14(2):117–8.
10. Kramer PF, Faraco Júnior IM, Meira R. A SEM investigation of accessory foramina in the furcation areas of primary molars. J Clin Pediatr Dent. 2003;27(2):157–61.
11. Gordon MPJ, Chandler NP. Electronic apex locators. Int Endod J. 2004;37(7):425–37.
12. Tchaou WS, Turng BF, Minah GE, Coll JA. In vitro inhibition of bacteria from root canals of primary teeth by various dental materials. Pediatr Dent. 1995;17(5):351–5.
13. Dummett Jr CO, Kopel H. Pediatric endodontics. In: Ingle J, editor. Endodontics. Philadelphia: Lea & Febiger; 2002. p. 861–902.
14. Fuks AB, Eidelman E, Pauker N. Root fillings with Endoflas in primary teeth: a retrospective study. J Clin Pediatr Dent. 2002;27(1):41–5.
15. Allen KR. Endodontic treatment of primary teeth. Aust Dent J. 1979;24(5):347–51.
16. Coll JA, Josell S, Casper JS. Evaluation of a one-appointment formocresol pulpectomy technique for primary molars. Pediatr Dent. 1985;7(2):123–9.
17. Mesbahi M, Talei S, Mollaverdi F, Kadkhodaza M. Comparison of root canal system configuration in primary teeth. Res J Biol Sci. 2010;5(7):488–91.
18. Lugliè PF, Grabesu V, Spano G, Lumbau A. Accessory foramina in the furcation area of primary molars. A SEM investigation. Eur J Paediatr Dent. 2012;13(4):329–32.
19. Fuks AB, Guelmann M, Kupietzky A. Current developments in pulp therapy for primary teeth. Endod Top. 2010;23(1):50–72.
20. Siqueira JF, Rôças IN, Paiva SSM, Guimarães-Pinto T, Magalhães KM, Lima KC. Bacteriologic investigation of the effects of sodium hypochlorite and chlorhexidine during the endodontic treatment of teeth with apical periodontitis. Oral Surg Oral Med Oral Pathol Oral Radiol Endod. 2007;104(1):122–30.
21. Ercan E, Ozekinci T, Atakul F, Gül K. Antibacterial activity of 2% chlorhexidine gluconate and 5.25% sodium hypochlorite in infected root canal: in vivo study. J Endod. 2004;30(2):84–7.
22. Zehnder M. Root canal irrigants. J Endod. 2006;32(5):389–98.
23. Rodd HD, Waterhouse PJ, Fuks AB, Fayle SA, Moffat MA. Pulp therapy for primary molars. Int J Paediatr Dent. 2006;16 Suppl 1:15–23.
24. Mehdipour O, Kleier DJ, Averbach RE. Anatomy of sodium hypochlorite accidents. Compend Contin Educ Dent. 2007;28(10):544–6, 548, 550.
25. Goswami M, Chhabra N, Kumar G, Verma M, Chhabra A. Sodium hypochlorite dental accidents. Paediatr Int Child Health. 2014;34(1):66–9.
26. Klein U, Kleier DJ. Sodium hypochlorite accident in a pediatric patient. Pediatr Dent. 2013;35(7):534–8.
27. Zhu W, Gyamfi J, Niu L, et al. Anatomy of sodium hypochlorite accidents involving facial ecchymosis – a review. J Dent. 2013;41(11):935–48.
28. Fedorowicz Z, Nasser M, Sequeira-Byron P, de Souza RF, Carter B, Heft M. Irrigants for non-surgical root canal treatment in mature permanent teeth. Cochrane Database Syst Rev. 2012;(9):CD008948.

29. Fuks AB, Eidelman E. Pulp therapy in the primary dentition. Curr Opin Dent. 1991;1(5):556–63.
30. Mortazavi M, Mesbahi M. Comparison of zinc oxide and eugenol, and Vitapex for root canal treatment of necrotic primary teeth. Int J Paediatr Dent. 2004;14(6):417–24.
31. Ozalp N, Saroğlu I, Sönmez H. Evaluation of various root canal filling materials in primary molar pulpectomies: an in vivo study. Am J Dent. 2005;18(6):347–50.
32. Siqueira JF, Lopes HP. Mechanisms of antimicrobial activity of calcium hydroxide: a critical review. Int Endod J. 1999;32(5):361–9.
33. Barja-Fidalgo F, Moutinho-Ribeiro M, Oliveira MAA, de Oliveira BH. A systematic review of root canal filling materials for deciduous teeth: is there an alternative for zinc oxide-eugenol? ISRN Dent. 2011;2011:367318.
34. Reddy S, Ramakrishna Y. Evaluation of antimicrobial efficacy of various root canal filling materials used in primary teeth: a microbiological study. J Clin Pediatr Dent. 2007;31(3):193–8.
35. Subramaniam P, Gilhotra K. Endoflas, zinc oxide eugenol and metapex as root canal filling materials in primary molars--a comparative clinical study. J Clin Pediatr Dent. 2011; 35(4):365–9.
36. Tchaou WS, Turng BF, Minah GE, Coll JA. Inhibition of pure cultures of oral bacteria by root canal filling materials. Pediatr Dent. 1996;18(7):444.
37. Kubota K, Golden BE, Penugonda B. Root canal filling materials for primary teeth: a review of the literature. ASDC J Dent Child. 1992;59(3):225–7.
38. Chen J-W, Jorden M. Materials for primary tooth pulp treatment: the present and the future. Endod Top. 2010;23(1):41–9.
39. Rifkin A. The root canal treatment of abscessed primary teeth--a three to four year follow-up. ASDC J Dent Child. 1982;49(6):428–31.
40. Garcia-Godoy F. Evaluation of an iodoform paste in root canal therapy for infected primary teeth. ASDC J Dent Child. 1987;54(1):30–4.
41. Rifkin A. A simple, effective, safe technique for the root canal treatment of abscessed primary teeth. ASDC J Dent Child. 1980;47(6):435–41.
42. Sadrian R, Coll JA. A long-term followup on the retention rate of zinc oxide eugenol filler after primary tooth pulpectomy. Pediatr Dent. 1993;15(4):249–53.
43. Barker BC, Lockett BC. Endodontic experiments with resorbable paste. Aust Dent J. 1971;16(6):364–72.
44. Primosch RE, Glomb TA, Jerrell RG. Primary tooth pulp therapy as taught in predoctoral pediatric dental programs in the United States. Pediatr Dent. 1997;19(2):118–22.
45. Dunston B, Coll JA. A survey of primary tooth pulp therapy as taught in US dental schools and practiced by diplomates of the American Board Of Pediatric Dentistry. Pediatr Dent. 2008;30(1):42–8.
46. Barcelos R, Santos MPA, Primo LG, Luiz RR, Maia LC. ZOE paste pulpectomies outcome in primary teeth: a systematic review. J Clin Pediatr Dent. 2011;35(3):241–8.
47. Nurko C, Ranly DM, García-Godoy F, Lakshmyya KN. Resorption of a calcium hydroxide/iodoform paste (Vitapex) in root canal therapy for primary teeth: a case report. Pediatr Dent. 2000;22(6):517–20.
48. Hegde S, Lala PK, Dinesh RB, Shubha AB. An in vitro evaluation of antimicrobial efficacy of primary root canal filling materials. J Clin Pediatr Dent. 2012;37(1):59–64.
49. Mass E, Zilberman UL. Endodontic treatment of infected primary teeth, using Maisto's paste. ASDC J Dent Child. 1989;56(2):117–20.
50. Reddy VV, Fernandes. Clinical and radiological evaluation of zinc oxide-eugenol and Maisto's paste as obturating materials in infected primary teeth--nine months study. J Indian Soc Pedod Prev Dent. 1996;14(2):39–44.
51. Holan G, Fuks AB. A comparison of pulpectomies using ZOE and KRI paste in primary molars: a retrospective study. Pediatr Dent. 1993;15(6):403–7.
52. Wright KJ, Barbosa SV, Araki K, Spångberg LS. In vitro antimicrobial and cytotoxic effects of Kri 1 paste and zinc oxide-eugenol used in primary tooth pulpectomies. Pediatr Dent. 1994;16(2):102–6.

53. Mente J, Seidel J, Buchalla W, Koch MJ. Electronic determination of root canal length in primary teeth with and without root resorption. Int Endod J. 2002;35(5):447–52.
54. Kielbassa AM, Muller U, Munz I, Monting JS. Clinical evaluation of the measuring accuracy of ROOT ZX in primary teeth. Oral Surg Oral Med Oral Pathol Oral Radiol Endod. 2003;95(1):94–100.
55. Beltrame APCA, Triches TC, Sartori N, Bolan M. Electronic determination of root canal working length in primary molar teeth: an in vivo and ex vivo study. Int Endod J. 2011;44(5):402–6.
56. Silva LAB, Leonardo MR, Nelson-Filho P, Tanomaru JMG. Comparison of rotary and manual instrumentation techniques on cleaning capacity and instrumentation time in deciduous molars. J Dent Child (Chic). 2004;71(1):45–7.
57. Canoglu H, Tekcicek MU, Cehreli ZC. Comparison of conventional, rotary, and ultrasonic preparation, different final irrigation regimens, and 2 sealers in primary molar root canal therapy. Pediatr Dent. 2006;28(6):518–23.
58. Crespo S, Cortes O, Garcia C, Perez L. Comparison between rotary and manual instrumentation in primary teeth. J Clin Pediatr Dent. 2008;32(4):295–8.
59. Pinheiro SL, Araujo G, Bincelli I, Cunha R, Bueno C. Evaluation of cleaning capacity and instrumentation time of manual, hybrid and rotary instrumentation techniques in primary molars. Int Endod J. 2012;45(4):379–85.
60. Seraj B, Ramezani G, Ghadimi S, Mosharrafian SH, Motahhary P, Safari M. In-vitro comparison of instrumentation time and cleaning capacity between endodontic handpiece and manual preparation techniques in primary molar teeth. Minerva Stomatol. 2013;62(1 – 2):17–22.
61. Ochoa-Romero T, Mendez-Gonzalez V, Flores-Reyes H, Pozos-Guillen AJ. Comparison between rotary and manual techniques on duration of instrumentation and obturation times in primary teeth. J Clin Pediatr Dent. 2011;35(4):359–63.
62. Miles JJ, Bulek AM, Cole DK, et al. Genetic and structural basis for selection of a ubiquitous T cell receptor deployed in Epstein-Barr virus infection. PLoS Pathog. 2010;6(11):1–15.
63. Barr ES, Kleier DJ, Barr NV. Use of nickel-titanium rotary files for root canal preparation in primary teeth. Pediatr Dent. 2000;22(1):77–8.
64. Soares F, Varella CH, Pileggi R, Adewumi A, Guelmann M. Impact of Er, Cr:YSGG laser therapy on the cleanliness of the root canal walls of primary teeth. J Endod. 2008;34(4):474–7.
65. Katz A, Mass E, Kaufman AY. Electronic apex locator: a useful tool for root canal treatment in the primary dentition. ASDC J Dent Child. 1996;63(6):414–7.
66. Oznurhan F, Ünal M, Kapdan A, Ozturk C, Aksoy S. Clinical evaluation of apex locator and radiography in primary teeth. Int J Paediatr Dent. 2015;25(3):199–203.
67. Topaloglu-Ak A, Aykut Yetkiner A, Güniz Baksi B, Eronat C. Ex vivo comparison of radiographic and electronic root canal length measurements in primary molars. Eur J Paediatr Dent. 2015;16(2):149–53.
68. Ahmad IA, Pani SC. Accuracy of electronic apex locators in primary teeth: a meta-analysis. Int Endod J. 2015;48(3):298–307.
69. Damle SG, Nadkarni UM. Calcium hydroxide and zinc oxide eugenol as root canal filling materials in primary molars: a comparative study. Aust Endod J. 2005;31(3):114–9.
70. Mani SA, Chawla HS, Tewari A, Goyal A. Evaluation of calcium hydroxide and zinc oxide eugenol as root canal filling materials in primary teeth. ASDC J Dent Child. 2000;67(2):142–7, 83.
71. Trairatvorakul C, Chunlasikaiwan S. Success of pulpectomy with zinc oxide-eugenol vs calcium hydroxide/iodoform paste in primary molars: a clinical study. Pediatr Dent. 2008; 30(4):303–8.
72. Jokinen MA, Kotilainen R, Poikkeus P, Poikkeus R, Sarkki L. Clinical and radiographic study of pulpectomy and root canal therapy. Scand J Dent Res. 1978;86(5):366–73.
73. Flaitz CM, Barr ES, Hicks MJ. Radiographic evaluation of pulpal therapy for primary anterior teeth. ASDC J Dent Child. 1989;56(3):182–5.
74. Barr ES, Flatiz CM, Hicks MJ. A retrospective radiographic evaluation of primary molar pulpectomies. Pediatr Dent. 1991;13(1):4–9.

75. Yacobi R, Kenny DJ, Judd PL, Johnston DH. Evolving primary pulp therapy techniques. J Am Dent Assoc. 1991;122(2):83–5.
76. Payne RG, Kenny DJ, Johnston DH, Judd PL. Two-year outcome study of zinc oxide-eugenol root canal treatment for vital primary teeth. J Can Dent Assoc. 1993;59(6):528–30, 533–6.
77. Primosch RE, Ahmadi A, Setzer B, Guelmann M. A retrospective assessment of zinc oxide-eugenol pulpectomies in vital maxillary primary incisors successfully restored with composite resin crowns. Pediatr Dent. 2005;27(6):470–7.
78. Moskovitz M, Sammara E, Holan G. Success rate of root canal treatment in primary molars. J Dent. 2005;33(1):41–7.
79. Coll JA, Josell S, Nassof S, Shelton P, Richards MA. An evaluation of pulpal therapy in primary incisors. Pediatr Dent. 1988;10(3):178–84.
80. Reyes AD, Reina ES. Root canal treatment in necrotic primary molars. J Pedod. 1989;14(1):36–9.
81. Thomas AM, Chandra S, Pandey RK. Elimination of infection in pulpectomized deciduous teeth: a short-term study using iodoform paste. J Endod. 1994;20(5):233–5.
82. Smaïl-Faugeron V, Courson F, Durieux P, Muller-Bolla M, Glenny A-M, Fron Chabouis H. Pulp treatment for extensive decay in primary teeth. Cochrane Database Syst Rev. 2014;8:CD003220.
83. Rewal N, Thakur AS, Sachdev V, Mahajan N. Comparison of endoflas and zinc oxide eugenol as root canal filling materials in primary dentition. J Indian Soc Pedod Prev Dent. 2014;32(4):317–21.
84. Cope A, Francis N, Wood F, Mann MK, Chestnutt IG. Systemic antibiotics for symptomatic apical periodontitis and acute apical abscess in adults. Cochrane Database Syst Rev. 2014;6:CD010136.
85. Nagle D, Reader A, Beck M, Weaver J. Effect of systemic penicillin on pain in untreated irreversible pulpitis. Oral Surg Oral Med Oral Pathol Oral Radiol Endod. 2000;90(5):636–40.
86. Fouad AF, Rivera EM, Walton RE. Penicillin as a supplement in resolving the localized acute apical abscess. Oral Surg Oral Med Oral Pathol Oral Radiol Endod. 1996;81(5):590–5.
87. Colgan R, Powers JH. Appropriate antimicrobial prescribing: approaches that limit antibiotic resistance. Am Fam Physician. 2001;64(6):999–1004.
88. Moskovitz M, Tickotsky N, Ashkar H, Holan G. Degree of root resorption after root canal treatment with iodoform-containing filling material in primary molars. Quintessence Int. 2012;43(5):361–8.
89. Haralabakis NB, Yiagtzis SC, Toutountzakis NM. Premature or delayed exfoliation of deciduous teeth and root resorption and formation. Angle Orthod. 1994;64(2):151–7.
90. Jerrell RG, Ronk SL. Developmental arrest of a succedaneous tooth following pulpectomy in a primary tooth. J Pedod. 1982;6(4):337–42.
91. Tannure PN, Fidalgo TK, Barcelos R, Gleiser R, Primo LG. Ectopic eruption of permanent incisors after predecessor pulpectomy: five cases. Gen Dent. 2011;59(4):e162–7.
92. Moskovitz M, Yahav D, Tickotsky N, Holan G. Long-term follow up of root canal treated primary molars. Int J Paediatr Dent. 2010;20(3):207–13.
93. Petel R, Moskovitz M, Tickotsky N, Halabi A, Goldstein J, Houri-Haddad Y. Cytotoxicity and proliferative effects of Iodoform-containing root canal-filling material on RAW 264.7 macrophage and RKO epithelial cell lines. Arch Oral Biol. 2013;58:75–81.
94. Rimondini L, Baroni C. Morphologic criteria for root canal treatment of primary molars undergoing resorption. Endod Dent Traumatol. 1995;11(3):136–41.
95. Weiss EI, Shalhav M, Fuss Z. Assessment of antibacterial activity of endodontic sealers by a direct contact test. Endod Dent Traumatol. 1996;12(4):179–84.
96. Nurko C, Garcia-Godoy F. Evaluation of a calcium hydroxide/iodoform paste (Vitapex) in root canal therapy for primary teeth. J Clin Pediatr Dent. 1999;23(4):289–94.
97. Geetha Priya PR, John JB, Elango I. Turner's hypoplasia and non-vitality: a case report of sequelae in permanent tooth. Contemp Clin Dent. 2010;1(4):251–4.
98. Ramar K, Mungara J. Clinical and radiographic evaluation of pulpectomies using three root canal filling materials: an in-vivo study. J Indian Soc Pedod Prev Dent. 2010;28(1):25–9.

Restoration of Pulp-Treated Teeth

7

Kevin J. Donly and Jungyi Alexis Liu

Contents

7.1 Introduction

The restoration of pulpally treated teeth is critical for the longitudinal success of maintaining the teeth within the oral cavity. There are a number of factors when choosing a restoration following pulp therapy such as the position of the tooth within the dental arch, which dictates the masticatory forces expected, as well as esthetics desired upon final restoration. The amount of tooth structure remaining

K.J. Donly, DDS, MS (✉) • J.A. Liu, DDS, MS
Department of Developmental Dentistry School of Dentistry, University of Texas Health Science Center at San Antonio, 7703 Floyd Curl Drive, San Antonio, TX 78229, USA
e-mail: donly@uthscsa.edu; liuja@uthscsa.edu

A.B. Fuks, B. Peretz (eds.), *Pediatric Endodontics: Current Concepts in Pulp Therapy for Primary and Young Permanent Teeth*,
DOI 10.1007/978-3-319-27553-6_7

after caries removal is important, and the clinician must remember that the clinical crown of the tooth becomes much more brittle after pulp therapy.

Unfortunately, there are no well-controlled prospective randomized clinical trials that compare full-coverage crown restorations following pulp treatment in the primary dentition. There are very few studies that have compared crowns when not being used subsequent to pulp therapy in the primary anterior and posterior dentitions. Therefore, we rely on extrapolated data, primarily from retrospective studies and case reports, to make the best restorative decision we can with the limited information available.

Clearly, there is a great need for more randomized clinical trials, which are hard to implement in a very young-aged population due to financial, behavioral, and social barriers. This chapter will discuss the possible restorations that may be placed following pulp therapy, the rationale for each type of restoration and the evidence that is available to support the use of various restorations.

7.2 Anterior Restorations (Primary Dentition)

7.2.1 Stainless Steel Crowns

Anterior stainless steel crowns have been recommended for many years to restore badly broken down teeth and teeth that have had pulp treatment, making them more sustainable to prevent tooth fracture [1]. These full-coverage crowns are indicated for patients exhibiting caries on multiple tooth surfaces, teeth that have dental caries extending to the incisal edge, teeth that have received pulp therapy, teeth that have extensive cervical caries or enamel demineralization, and teeth that are difficult to isolate due to the extent of caries or subsequent to the poor behavior of a very young child during treatment [2]. The anterior stainless steel crowns are resistant to fracture, have excellent wear characteristics, and can be crimped at the gingival margin to be retained to the tooth, even if there is minimal tooth structure remaining. Although these anterior stainless steel crowns provide a very stable restoration, the main disadvantage is the silver color that many children and/or their parents find dissatisfying. The open-face stainless steel crown technique, where the metal on the facial surface of the crown is removed and a tooth-colored resin is placed, can provide a better esthetic appearance (Fig. 7.1).

7.2.2 Pre-veneered Stainless Steel Crowns

Pre-veneered stainless steel crowns were introduced into the market place to offer a more esthetic anterior restoration, compared to the typical stainless steel crown, when restoring primary anterior teeth [3]. Again, this full-coverage restoration provided the strength to maintain teeth that had extensive caries and multiple tooth surface involvement and teeth which required pulp therapy yet presented an esthetic facial surface upon cementation. The preparation design for the pre-veneered stainless steel crown is more aggressive than the preparation for strip crowns, but provides the opportunity to achieve an esthetic restoration when isolation of the tooth is difficult to place strip crowns. The main problem with these types of crowns was the possibility of fracture to all or part of the resin facing on the crowns. If there is a chip or break in the white facing, it is difficult to repair (Fig. 7.2). Replacement with a new crown is usually needed to achieve a better esthetic result. Also, the crown cannot be crimped on the facial surface because this increases the fracture or partial fracture of the resin facing. Therefore, the crimp on the lingual surface of the tooth is relied upon for retention of the pre-veneered crowns. Uncooperative behavior of very young children may be a contraindication of the use of pre-veneered crowns because their crown preparations and crown fitting take additional time compared to the standard stainless steel crown.

When the literature was reviewed for an evidence-based assessment of anterior crowns for primary teeth [4], a small number of papers were referenced to evaluate the parental satisfaction and clinical success of resin-faced stainless steel crowns [5, 6].

Parents appeared to be satisfied with two different resin-faced crowns, even though 30–40 % of the crowns demonstrated partial or full resin facing loss in these reports. In another report, Champagne et al. indicated a 93 % parental satisfaction at a mean of 13 months post-crown placement [7]. In a retrospective study, MacLean et al. reported a 91 % success rate of anterior pre-veneered crowns over an average of 12.9 months following crown placement [8].

7.2.3 Strip Crowns

Resin-based composite strip crowns have been used as full-coverage restorations in the primary anterior dentition over the past four decades [2, 9]. Placement of resin into a prefabricated primary tooth celluloid form and placing it over a prepared tooth allows for full coverage and an excellent esthetic outcome [10]. There must be enough remaining tooth structure, or the tooth needs to have a resin or glass ionomer cement crown base placed, so there is adequate tooth structure to acid etch and bond for a successful restoration. Likewise, the prepared tooth must be isolated well to have a resin bond to prevent marginal microleakage.

Review of the literature identified three retrospective studies evaluating the clinical and radiographic success of strip crown restorations of the primary anterior dentition [11–13]. Kupietzky et al. evaluated 112 strip crown restorations in 40 children, which had been in place for an average of 18 months. None of the restorations were completely lost, and 12 % had some loss of resin-based composite material. This resulted in an 88 % overall retention of the strip crown [11]. Kupietzky et al. again retrospectively evaluated strip crown restorations. This included 145 strip crown restorations placed in 52 children, which had been in place for an average of 31.3 months. None of the restorations were completely lost, and 20 % had some loss of resin-based composite. This resulted in an 80 % overall retention of the strip crown. Radiographic assessment was also completed in this study. Two teeth revealed radiographic evidence of pupal pathology requiring treatment [12]. Ram and Fuks, in a retrospective study of 200 records of children aged 22–48 months that had returned for a follow-up appointment after at least 24 months, demonstrated more than 80 % of strip crowns were successful. They reported the number of carious tooth surfaces at baseline to influence the treatment outcome, with the failure rate being higher for primary central incisors which had formed carious tooth surfaces [13]. In general, studies showed a favorable success rate of strip crown retention over an 18-month to 31-month mean survival evaluation period.

More variable success rates were noted when strip crowns were being placed over teeth being restored when the child was being treated with the aid of general anesthesia, restorations being evaluated for retention at intervals from 6 months to 2 years [14–18]. O'Sullivan and Curzon reviewed 80 children treated under general anesthesia that has at least a 2-year follow-up. Sixteen strip crowns had been placed, and all of them were successful at the follow-up evaluation [14]. Su and Chen reviewed 38 cases where children received comprehensive dental care under general anesthesia and returned for a follow-up at least 1 year later. The authors reported a 22 % failure for the 50 strip crowns [15]. Eidelman et al. in a retrospective study that evaluated restoration success of 34 children treated under general anesthesia reported that 90 % of strip crowns were successful after 24 months compared to a 63 % success of strip crowns that were placed on children that were sedated [16]. Tate et al., in another retrospective study of 63 patients that had strip crowns placed when being treated under general anesthesia and returned for at least a 6-month postoperative evaluation, reported a 51 % failure rate of the strip crowns [17]. Al-Eheideb and Herman evaluated the dental records of 54 children treated under general anesthesia. On these patients, 23 strip crowns were placed. Return evaluations that ranged from 6 months to 27 months revealed a 30 % failure rate of the strip crowns [18]. An important note was the fact that Kupietzky et al. reported strip crowns discolored when placed over teeth that had a pulpectomy which was obturated with iodoform paste [11].

7.2.4 Zirconia Crowns

Zirconia crowns are relatively new in the practice of pediatric restorative dentistry [19–21].

These crowns are very strong and durable as well as esthetically pleasing (Fig. 7.3). The strength and esthetics of these crowns make them desirable for severely decayed teeth or pulpally treated teeth, where full coverage is beneficial.

Unfortunately, since these preformed crowns cannot be crimped, preparation design and perfect tooth isolation are relied upon to prevent contamination and provide the cement bond necessary for a successful restoration. Longitudinal studies will surely offer further information on the success of these zirconia crowns in pediatric dentistry.

7.3 Posterior Restorations (Primary Dentition)

7.3.1 Stainless Steel Crowns

Posterior stainless steel crowns have been the traditional restoration of choice for primary molars exhibiting severe caries, multiple surface caries, and teeth which had received pulp therapy [22–24]. The stainless steel crown provides full-coverage reinforcement of severely damaged teeth and those that become more fracture prone following pulp treatment (Fig. 7.4). It also seals the preparation margins to prevent marginal microleakage which can lead to restoration failure.

There have been a number of retrospective studies evaluating the long-term success of stainless steel crowns, comparing them to other restorative materials. Roberts et al. evaluated the survival of resin-modified glass ionomer cement and stainless steel crown restorations in primary molars [25]. They reported that stainless steel crowns were superior for larger restorations; however, resin-modified glass ionomer cement restorations were very successful when used as small class I or class II restoration. When stainless steel crowns were compared to amalgam restorations in the primary dentition, it was found that there is evidence that stainless steel crowns demonstrate greater longevity and reduced need for retreatment, compared to multi-surface amalgam restorations [26–31].

Another systematic review of the literature evaluated the longevity of occlusally stressed restorations in posterior primary teeth reporting that stain less steel crowns remain the desirable restoration for primary molars with multiple surface caries but also noted adhesive restorations were successful for smaller restorations [32].

A retrospective study evaluated the success rate of 141 molars that had been treated by pulpotomies and were restored with either amalgam or stainless steel crowns, with a follow-up ranging from 6 to 103 months [33]. The results indicated, with, that stainless steel crowns were preferable unless the amalgam restoration was only an occlusal one-surface restoration with natural tooth exfoliation within 2 years of restoration placement. Other studies have been published that retrospectively reported the success rates of pulpotomies and indirect pulp therapy which identified the restoration over the pulpotomy or indirect pulp therapy [33–37]. The studies indicated the placement of a stainless steel crown immediately after a pulpotomy or indirect pulp treatment significantly increased the survival of the tooth.

7.3.2 Pre-veneered Stainless Steel Crowns

Posterior pre-veneered stainless steel crowns are available for use as an esthetic restoration of primary molars. Two studies evaluated the clinical success of these pre-veneered stainless steel crowns. Leith et al. reported 81 % of resin facings were intact at 12 months and parents indicated satisfaction with the restorative crown [38]. The same authors recalled patients after 3 years and found 53 % of the veneer facings to be intact [39]. Again, parents indicated their satisfaction with the esthetic pre-veneered crowns.

Ram et al. reported a 4-year evaluation of ten conventional stainless steel crowns and ten pre-veneered stainless steel crowns [40]. At 4 years, all ten pre-veneered crowns had chipping of the resin; however, the crowns still performed intraorally very well and the periodontal health adjacent to all crowns was good.

Therefore, the pre-veneered stainless steel crowns can be an alternative to the conventional stainless steel crown, but chipping of the resin veneer facing can be expected. Marginal crimping on the facing of these crowns can compromise the resin facing, so tooth preparation to adapt to the crown size becomes more critical for crown retention.

7.3.3 Resin-Based Restorations

Although a majority of retrospective studies recommend the use of stainless steel crowns for the restoration of extensive caries or following pulp therapy, there are some that address the use of resin-based composites in these circumstances. Atieh completed a 2-year randomized clinical trial comparing stainless steel crowns and resin restorations (sandwich restoration with resin-modified glass ionomer cement covered by resin-based composite), for restored primary molars following pulpotomy treatment. There was no significant difference in success of stainless steel crowns and the resin-based restorations, both having greater than 90 % success [41].

Other studies indicated success of resin-based restorations for pulpotomized primary molars [42–45]. Zulfikaroglu et al., in a prospective 12-month randomized clinical trial of 75 restorations, reported an 81 % success of class II adhesive restorations in primary molars that had received pulpectomies [42]. In another clinical trial, 100 resin-based class II composite restorations and 100 polyacid-modified resin-based class II composite restorations in 84 children were evaluated at 24 months. Of the 80 resin-based composite restorations that were available at 24 months, 100 % were caries-free. Of the 72 polyacid-modified resin-based composite restorations available at 24 months, 97.2 % were caries-free. However, 2 % of resin-based composite restorations and 17 % of polyacid-modified resin-based composite restorations revealed radiographic evidence of root resorption or pericoronal bone resorption and were extracted [43]. Guelmann et al., in a literature review of two laboratory studies, three retrospective studies, and four prospective clinical trials, concluded adhesive resin-based composite restorations demonstrated promising results as an alternative restorative material to stainless steel crowns when restoring primary molars following pulpotomy treatment [44]. Caceda published a retrospective study that included the evaluation of 51 primary molars which had received pulpotomy treatment with subsequent class I or class II resin-based composite restorations. These restorations had been placed in children 2–11 years of age, and the evaluation time period ranged from 12 to 54 months. The reported results revealed that all 51 resin-based class I and class II restorations over the primary molars that had received pulpotomy treatment were successful [45].

In a retrospective study by Guelmann et al., which involved the radiographic assessment of primary molar pulpotomies restored with resin-based materials, it was concluded that restoration of pulpotomized primary molars with resin-based composite was inferior to reported success rates using stainless steel crowns [46].

Hutcheson et al. published the findings of a randomized, controlled trial comparing multi-surface resin-based composite and stainless steel crown restorations following mineral trioxide aggregate (MTA) pulpotomies. Although all restorations were successful at 12 months, the teeth restored with resin-based composite discolored and were not considered an esthetic alternative to stainless steel crowns [47].

7.3.4 Zirconia

Zirconia crowns are available for the restoration of primary molars (Fig. 7.5). These full-coverage posterior primary crowns can be used to restore teeth with severe caries and multi-surface caries and teeth that have received pulpal therapy. Isolation of the tooth is critical for the placement of zirconia crowns. Preparation design of slight occlusal convergence and isolation to keep the tooth dry for cement bonding are critical for clinical success. There is currently no published data of the use of posterior zirconia crowns with pulpal therapy or without pulpal therapy. Future studies will offer further information on the clinical success of the primary posterior zirconia crowns.

7.4 Restoration Outcomes on Children Treated Under General Anesthesia

Some children, due to extensive caries and uncooperative behavior associated with very young children or children with special healthcare needs, have dental care provided under general anesthesia. Retrospective studies on the outcomes of dental procedures performed on children under general anesthesia reported that stainless steel crowns are more likely to be successful and last longer than multi-surface amalgam or resin-based composite restorations [18, 48, 49]. Therefore, the American Academy of Pediatric Dentistry (AAPD) recommends the use of stainless steel crowns for severe caries and multi-surface caries and on teeth of children considered to be at high risk for the development of secondary caries [22, 24].

7.5 Posterior Restorations (Permanent Dentition)

The restoration of permanent molars following pulp treatment occurs in the practice of pediatric dentistry. Often, this is associated with teeth diagnosed with molar incisor hypomineralization (MIH). Following pulp treatment, these teeth were traditionally restored with full-coverage stainless steel crowns in the adolescent patient. Patients were instructed to have the stainless steel crown replaced with a gold crown, porcelain fused to metal crown, porcelain crown, or zirconia crown as the patient matured and had a fully erupted permanent dentition. The AAPD through a Pediatric Restorative Dentistry Symposium, recommends stainless steel crowns for adolescents that are in need of full coverage of permanent molars [24].

Zirconia crowns are now available in preprepared standardized custom sizes for permanent molars. These crowns can also be utilized and offer an esthetically pleasing restoration. Preparation for these crowns is provided by instructions from the manufacturer.

Case 7.1: Open-Face Stainless Steel Crowns for Primary Incisors

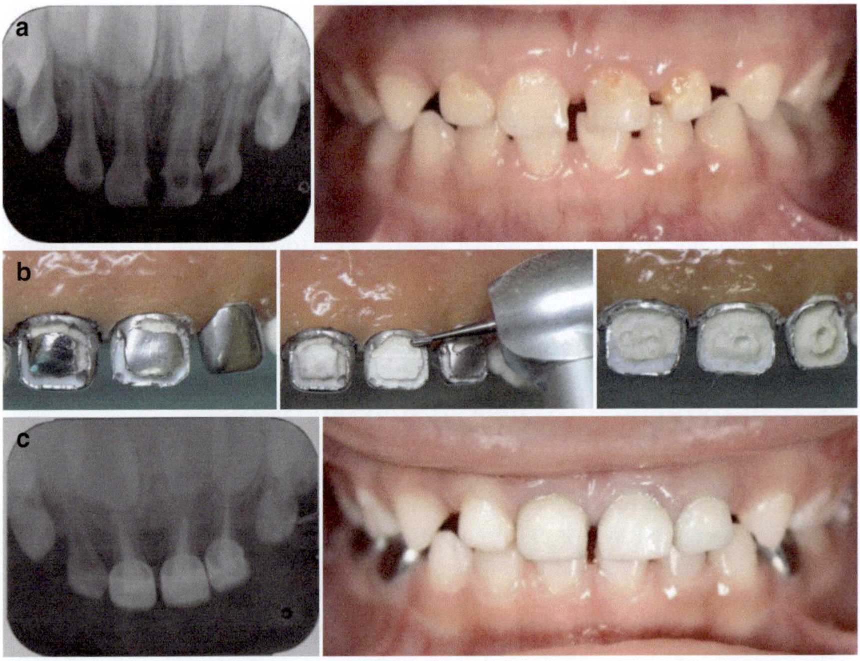

Fig. 7.1 (**a**) Maxillary right and left primary central incisors and maxillary left primary lateral incisor with deep caries and symptoms of pulpitis. (**b**) Illustration of the metal on the facial surface of the stainless steel crowns being removed with a 330 bur and undercuts being created to increase retention of the resin. (**c**) Pulpectomies were completed and stainless steel crowns were placed with the open window technique

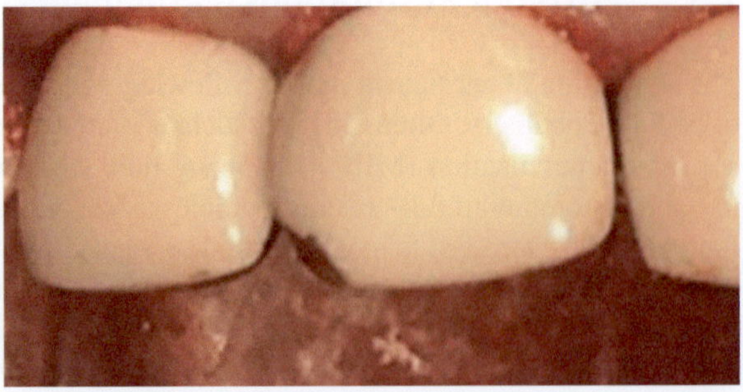

Fig. 7.2 A chip in the white facing of a pre-veneered crown on a primary maxillary right central incisor

Case 7.2: Zirconia Crowns for Primary Incisors

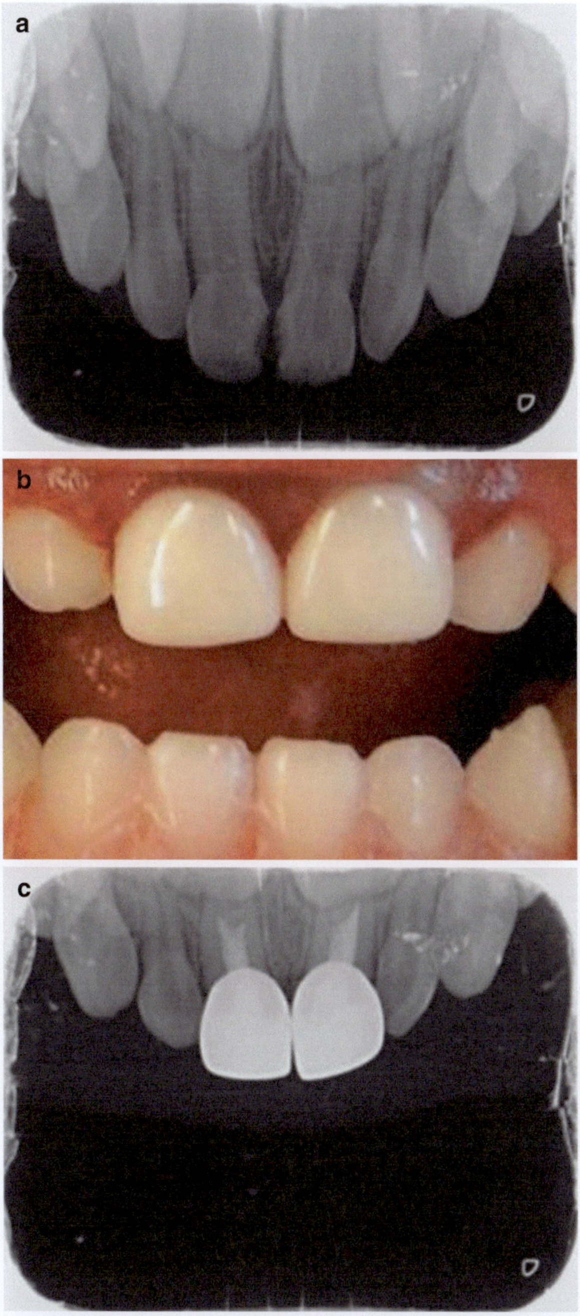

Fig. 7.3 Maxillary right and left primary central incisors with deep caries and symptoms of nocturnal pain. Pulpectomies were completed and zirconia crowns placed. (**a**) Pretreatment radiograph. (**b**) Intraoral photographs taken immediately after treatment. (**c**) Radiograph immediately after treatment (Photograph courtesy of Dr. Yi-Hsuan Liu)

Case 7.3: Stainless Steel Crowns for Primary Molars

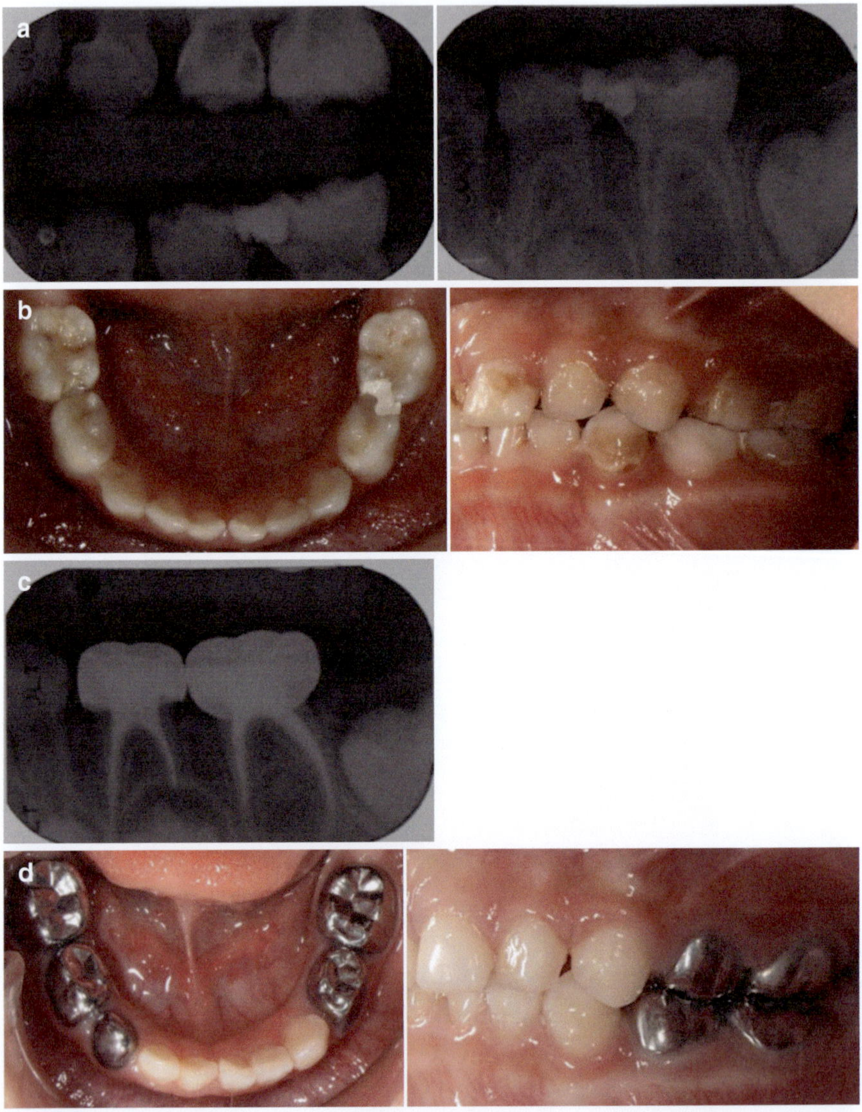

Fig. 7.4 (**a**) Mandibular left first and second primary molars with deep caries and the symptom of spontaneous pain. Pulpectomies were completed in a single appointment and stainless steel crowns were placed. (**b**) Pretreatment photographs. (**c**) Radiograph immediately after treatment. (**d**) Intraoral photographs taken after all treatment was completed

Case 7.4: Zirconia Crown for a Primary Molar

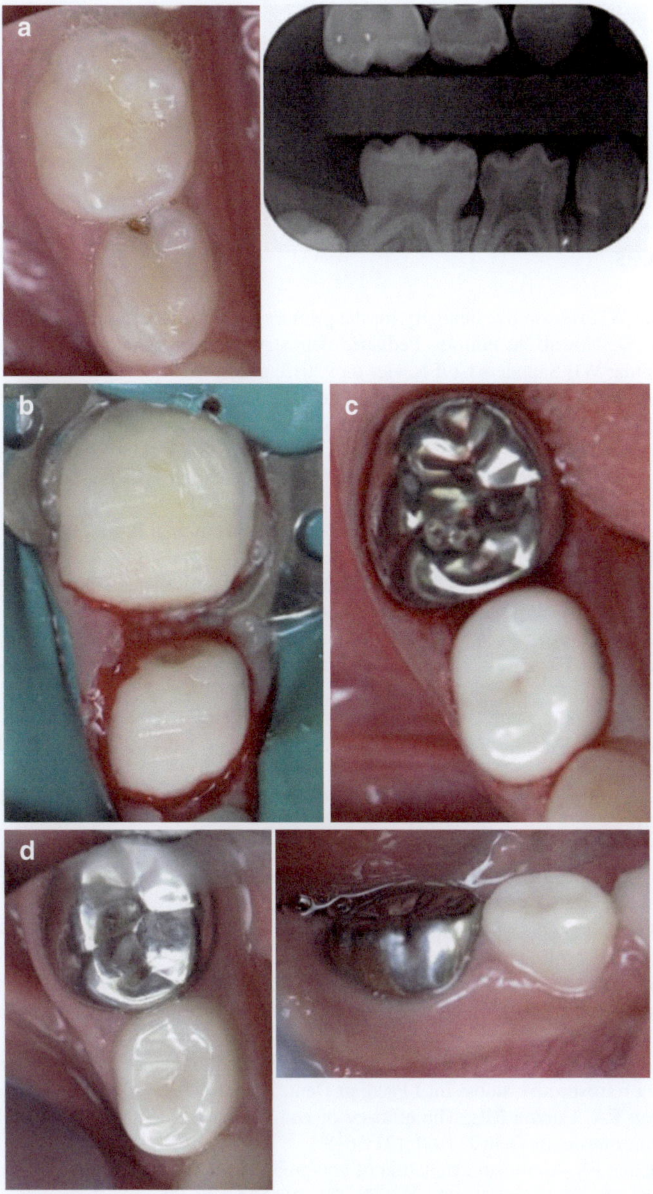

Fig. 7.5 (**a**) A preoperative photograph and a bitewing radiograph of an asymptomatic mandibular right first primary molar with deep caries. (**b**) Indirect pulp therapy was performed. Photograph taken after tooth preparation for a zirconia crown and before placing calcium hydroxide over the remaining carious dentin. (**c**) Intraoral photograph taken immediately after the tooth was restored with a zirconia crown. (**d**) A 12-month postoperative photograph of an indirect pulp treatment with a zirconia crown on the mandibular right first primary molar. (**e**) Postoperative bitewing radiograph taken at 12-month follow-up

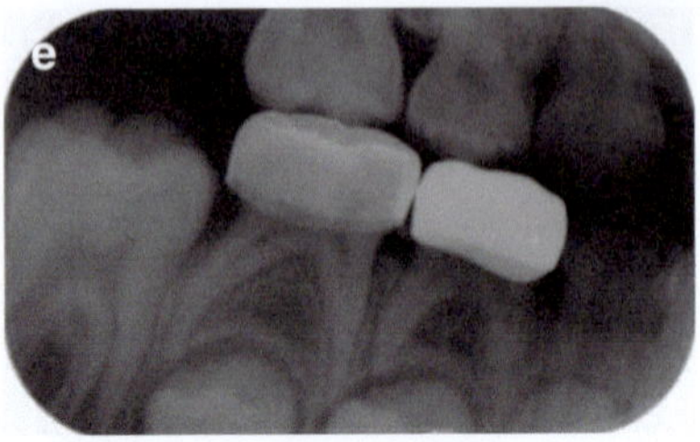

Fig. 7.5 (continued)

References

1. Waggoner WF. Restorative dentistry for the primary dentition. In: Casamassimo PS, Fields H, McTigue D, Nowak A, editors. Pediatric dentistry: infancy through adolescence. 5th ed. Philadelphia: WB Saunders Co/Elsevier Inc; 2013. p. 304–32.
2. Waggoner WF. Restoring primary anterior teeth. Pediatr Dent. 2002;24:511–6.
3. Croll TP, Helpin M. Preformed resin-veneered stainless steel crowns for restoration of primary incisors. Quintessence Int. 1996;27:309–13.
4. Waggoner WF. Anterior crowns for primary anterior teeth: an evidence based assessment of the literature. Eur Arch Paediatr Dent. 2006;7:53–7.
5. Roberts C, Lee JY, Wright JT. Clinical evaluation of and parental satisfaction with resin-faced stainless steel crowns. Pediatr Dent. 2001;23:28–31.
6. Shah PV, Lee JY, Wright JT. Clinical success and parental satisfaction with anterior preveneered primary stainless steel crowns. Pediatr Dent. 2004;26:391–5.
7. Champagne C, Waggoner WF, Ditmyer M, Casamassimo PS, MacLean J. Parental satisfaction with preveneered stainless steel crowns for primary anterior teeth. Pediatr Dent. 2007; 29:465–9.
8. MacLean JK, Champagne CE, Waggoner WF, Ditmyer MM, Casamassimo P. Clinical outcomes for primary teeth treated with preveneered stainless steel crowns. Pediatr Dent. 2007; 29:377–81.
9. Lee JK. Restoration of primary anterior teeth: review of the literature. Pediatr Dent. 2002; 24:506–10.
10. Webber DL, Epstein NB, Wong JW, Tsamtsouris A. A method of restoring primary anterior teeth within the aid of a celluloid crown form and composite resins. Pediatr Dent. 1979; 1:244–6.
11. Kupietzky A, Waggoner WF, Galea J. The clinical and radiographic success of bonded resin composite strip crowns for primary incisors. Pediatr Dent. 2003;25:77–8.
12. Kupietzky A, Waggoner WF, Galea J. Long-term photographic and radiographic assessment of bonded resin composite strip crowns for primary incisors: results after 3 years. Pediatr Dent. 2005;7:221–5.
13. Ram D, Fuks AB. Clinical performance of resin-bonded composite strip crowns in primary incisors: a retrospective study. Int J Paediatr Dent. 2006;16:49–54.
14. O'Sullivan EA, Curzon ME. The efficacy of comprehensive dental care for children under general anesthesia. Br Dent J. 1991;171:56–8.
15. Su HL, Chen PS. A clinical evaluation of comprehensive dental treatment for children under general anesthesia. Changgeng Yi Xue Za Zhi. 1992;15:188–92.
16. Eidelman E, Faibis S, Peretz B. A comparison of restorations for children with early childhood caries treated under general anesthesia or conscious sedation. Pediatr Dent. 2000;22:33–7.
17. Tate AR, Ng MW, Needleman HL, Acs G. Failure rates of restorative procedures following dental rehabilitation under general anesthesia. Pediatr Dent. 2002;24:69–71.
18. Al-Eheideb AA, Herman NG. Outcomes of dental procedures performed on children under general anesthesia. J Clin Pediatr Dent. 2003;27:181–4.

19. Karaca S, Ozbay G, Kargul B. Primary zirconia crown restorations for children with early childhood caries. Acta Stomatol Croatica. 2013;47:64–71.
20. Planells del Pozo P, Fuks AB. Zirconia crowns – an esthetic and resistant restorative alternative for ECC affected primary teeth. J Clin Pediatr Dent. 2014;38:193–5.
21. Waggoner WF. Restoring primary anterior teeth: updated for 2014. Pediatr Dent. 2015;37:163–70.
22. Seale NS. The use of stainless steel crowns. Pediatr Dent. 2002;24:501–5.
23. Randall RC. Preformed metal crowns for primary and permanent teeth: review of the literature. Pediatr Dent. 2002;24:489–500.
24. Seale NS, Randall R. The use of stainless steel crowns: a systematic literature review. Pediatr Dent. 2015;37:147–62.
25. Roberts JF, Attari N, Sherriff M. The survival of resin modified glass ionomer and stainless steel crown restorations in primary molars placed in a specialist pediatric dental practice. Br Dent J. 2005;198:427–31.
26. Randall RC, Vrijhoef MMA, Wilson NHF. Efficacy of preformed metal crowns vs amalgam restorations in primary molar teeth: a systematic review. J Am Dent Assoc. 2000;131: 337–43.
27. Messer LB, Levering NJ. The durability of primary molar restorations: II. Observations and predictions of success of stainless steel crowns. Pediatr Dent. 1988;10:81–5.
28. Levering NJ, Messer LB. The durability of primary molar restorations: I. Observations and predictions of success of amalgams. Pediatr Dent. 1988;10:74–80.
29. Levering NJ, Messer LB. The durability of primary molar restorations: III. Costs associated with placement and replacement. Pediatr Dent. 1988;10:86–93.
30. Attari N, Roberts JF. Restoration of primary teeth with crowns: a systematic review of the literature. Eur Arch Paediatr Dent. 2006;7:58–63.
31. Mata AF, Bebermeyer RD. Stainless steel crowns versus amalgams in the primary dentition and decision- making in clinical practice. Gen Dent. 2006;54:347–50.
32. Hickel R, Kaaden C, Paschos E, Buerkle V, Garcia-Godoy F, Manhart J. Longevity of occlusally-stressed restoration s in posterior primary teeth. Am J Dent. 2005;18:198–211.
33. Holan G, Fuks AB, Keltz N. Success rate of formocresol pulpotomy in primary molars restored with stainless steel crown vs amalgam. Pediatr Dent. 2002;24:212–6.
34. Farooq NS, Coll JA, Kuwabara A, Shelton P. Success rates of formocresol pulpotomy and indirect pulp therapy in the treatment of deep dentinal caries in primary teeth. Pediatr Dent. 2000;22:278–86.
35. Al-Zayer MA, Straffon LH, Feigal RJ, Welch KB. Indirect pulp treatment of primary posterior teeth: a retrospective study. Pediatr Dent. 2003;25:29–36.
36. Guelmann M, Fair J, Bimstein E. Permanent versus temporary restorations after emergency pulpotomies in primary molars. Pediatr Dent. 2005;27:478–81.
37. Moskovitz M, Sammara E, Holan G. Stainless steel crowns improve success rate of root canal treatment in primary teeth. J Dent. 2005;33:41–7.
38. Leith R, O'Connell AC. A clinical study evaluating success of two commercially available preveneered primary molar stainless steel crowns. Pediatr Dent. 2011;33:300–6.
39. O'Connell AC, Kratunova E, Leith R. Posterior preveneered stainless steel crowns: clinical performance after three years. Pediatr Dent. 2014;36:254–8.
40. Ram D, Fuks AB, Eidelman E. Long-term clinical performance of esthetic primary molar crowns. Pediatr Dent. 2003;25:582–4.
41. Atieh M. Stainless steel crown versus modified open-sandwich restorations for primary molars: a two- year randomized clinical trial. Int J Paediatr Dent. 2008;18:325–32.
42. Zulfikaroglu BT, Atac AS, Cehreli ZC. Clinical performance of class II adhesive restorations in pulpectomized primary molars: 1 2-month results. J Dent Child. 2008;75:33–43.
43. Cehreli ZC, Centinguc A, Cengiz SB, Altay AN. Clinical performance of pulpotomized primary molars restored with resin-based materials. 24-month results. Am J Dent. 2006;19:262–6.
44. Guelmann M, Shapira J, Silva DR, Fuks AB. Esthetic restorative options for pulpotomized primary molars: a review of literature. J Clin Pediatr Dent. 2011;36:123–6.

45. Caceda JH. The use of resin-based composite restorations in pulpotomized primary molars. J Dent Child. 2007;74:147–50.
46. Guelmann M, Mcllwain MF, Primosch RE. Radiographic assessment of primary molar pulpotomies restored with resin-based materials. Pediatr Dent. 2005;27:24–7.
47. Hutcheson C, Seale NS, McWhorter A, Kerins C, Wright J. Multi-surface composite vs stainless steel crown restorations after mineral trioxide aggregate pulpotomy: a randomized controlled trial. Pediatr Dent. 2012;34:460–7.
48. Drummond BK, Davidson LE, Williams SM, Moffat SM, Ayers KM. Outcomes two, three and four years after comprehensive care under general anesthesia. N Z Dent J. 2004;100:32–7.
49. Sheller B, Williams BJ, Hays K, Mancl L. Reasons for repeat dental treatment under general anesthesia for the healthy child. Pediatr Dent. 2003;25:546–52.

Pulp Therapy for the Young Permanent Dentition

8

Eyal Nuni

Contents

Pulp injury caused by caries or trauma is still commonly found in the young permanent dentition. Young permanent teeth in which root development and apical closure have not been completed are termed immature teeth. After apical closure, these teeth are classified as mature teeth [1].

E. Nuni, DMD
Department of Endodontics, Hadassah School of Dental Medicine, Hebrew University, 12272, Jerusalem, Israel
e-mail: eyal@drnuni.com

A.B. Fuks, B. Peretz (eds.), *Pediatric Endodontics: Current Concepts in Pulp Therapy for Primary and Young Permanent Teeth*,
DOI 10.1007/978-3-319-27553-6_8

Pulp necrosis in an immature permanent tooth will lead to a compromised prognosis and a potential for premature tooth loss. Endodontic treatment for these teeth present several challenges and will be described further in this chapter [2, 3].

Therefore the aim of all treatment planning for young permanent teeth is to preserve pulp vitality, providing conditions for continuous root development and physiologic dentin apposition.

8.1 The Pulp-Dentin Complex in Young Permanent Teeth

Similarly to what was described for primary teeth (see Chap. 3) the most important and most difficult aspect of pulp therapy is determining the health of the pulp or its stage of inflammation. Young permanent teeth have a highly cellular pulp and a rich vascular supply providing a better healing potential than the same teeth in adults. The degree of root development of these teeth will affect the considerations in determining the treatment plan [1].

As in primary teeth, tertiary dentin is produced as a reaction of the pulp to caries and operative procedures also in young permanent teeth (see Chaps. 2 and 4).

The dentin matrix is considered to be a reservoir of bioactive molecules and growth factors, sequestered during dentinogenesis. During dental tissue injury (i.e., caries and bacterial acid secretion) these molecules may be released from the dentin with other components of the extracellular matrix, inducing the formation of tertiary dentin. Members of the transforming growth factor superfamily, specifically TGF-βs, have received considerable attention in effecting mesenchymal cells and inducing dentin regeneration [4, 5]. These bioactive molecules are hypothesized to provide the signals involved in the recruitment of the progenitor stem cells to the site of pulp injury, and their proliferation and differentiation in order to initiate tissue regeneration and dentin bridge formation (see Chap. 2).

Pulp exposures in young permanent teeth are mainly due either to caries or trauma. In carious exposures the pulp and the dentin are infected, whereas in iatrogenic exposures during operative procedures only the dentin may be infected and the pulp may sometimes not even be inflamed. In traumatic pulp exposures the dentin is not infected, and the pulp tissue may remain vital and not infected if treated soon after the injury [1].

8.2 Clinical Pulpal Diagnosis in Young Permanent Teeth

Clinical pulpal diagnosis in the young permanent dentition is similar to that of primary teeth (see Chap. 3). This section will emphasize the differences between primary and young permanent teeth. Determining the nature and extent of pulpal inflammation is a key factor in achieving an appropriate treatment plan. However, the clinician should bear in mind that correlation between the pulp status and the clinical signs and symptoms is very limited [6].

8.2.1 Medical and Dental History

Medical and dental history should always be carefully documented, followed by a thorough clinical and radiographic examinations. In cases of trauma, both patient and parents should be asked about the timing and nature of the injury, and whether previous treatment or traumatic incidents have occurred.

As described in Chap. 3 provoked pain is usually triggered by a thermal or osmotic stimulus (e.g., cold, sweet) and ceases when the stimulus is removed, while spontaneous pain is not associated with an external stimulus, may arise at any time of the day, or wake the child from sleep. Spontaneous pain and/or provoked pain which continues long after the stimulus is removed (over shoot) are usually associated with extensive, irreversible pulpal inflammation extending into the root canals. Although in primary teeth pulpectomy is the treatment of choice in this cases, immature permanent teeth should be carefully considered for pulpotomy, apexogenesis, or even regenerative treatment because of the destructive nature of losing vital pulp functions.

8.2.2 Clinical Examination

Clinical examination should comprise both careful extraoral and intraoral examinations. Extra oral examination should focus on the presence of swelling, local lymphadenopathy and extra oral sinus tracts. Intraoral examination should assess the tooth suspected as the origin of pain, but also all the teeth on the same side should be inspected carefully, as referred pain can occur. The presence of extra oral or intraoral sinus tract requires the performance of a tracing radiograph in order to disclose the origin of the infection. Tooth discoloration is also an important finding especially in traumatized teeth [1]. Similarly to what occurs in primary teeth, thermal and electric pulp test (EPT) sensibility tests have limited reliability in young permanent teeth, and do not reflect the extent of pulp inflammation [7, 8]. Studies concluded that until innervation is completed (after 4–5 years in function) the EPT is not a reliable means of determining tooth vitality [9]. Cold test has been found more reliable in immature permanent teeth [7, 8]. Reliability of sensibility tests in traumatized teeth, especially in the period adjacent to the traumatic incident is limited, because of possible damage to the pulp innervation system [10].

Sensitivity to percussion does not indicate the state of the pulp inflammation but is rather an indication of inflammation in the periodontal ligament (PDL). This inflammation is most often a result of pulp inflammation that extended into the PDL or a sequel of dental trauma [1].

Pulp diagnosis is based upon the integration of the history and the clinical examination, but cannot be verified histologically. Thus, for practical reasons the state of the pulp is classified as reversible (treatable) or irreversible (untreatable) pulpitis [11]. Diagnosis of reversible pulpitis indicates that the inflammation can subside, and vital pulp therapy is a potential treatment option. Vital pulp treatment options range from indirect pulp treatment, direct pulp capping and partial or cervical pulpotomy, depending on the progress of the inflammatory process within the pulp and the degree of root development.

Clinically, the difference between reversible and irreversible pulpitis is frequently determined on the basis of the duration and intensity of the pain sensation. Over shoot to cold stimuli, spontaneous pain or referred pain will lead to a diagnosis of irreversible or untreatable pulpitis. As mentioned, although in primary teeth pulpectomy is the treatment of choice in these cases, immature permanent teeth should be carefully considered for pulpotomy, apexogenesis, or regenerative treatment, in an attempt to enable further tooth development.

8.2.3 Radiographic Examination

Good quality radiographs should complement a careful clinical examination. Bite-wing radiographs are necessary for assessing the depth of caries lesions, the morphology of the pulp chamber, the height of the pulp horns, the integrity and depth of restorations and the level of bone support (Fig. 8.1a). Bite-wing can also demonstrate the presence of a calcified bridge in the pulp chamber indicating the formation of tertiary dentin by a vital pulp in response to caries or pulp treatment.

Periapical radiographs should be inspected for continuity of the periodontal ligament in order to diagnose inflammatory and resorptive lesions. The interpretation of radiographs of young, immature permanent teeth can be difficult, due to their normally large and open apex and radiolucent apical papilla. Less experienced dentists treating these teeth should avoid confusing pathologic changes with normal apical anatomy [1]. In a young child a vertical bite-wing with a small size radiograph can be used instead of a periapical radiograph in order to see the periapical area of posterior teeth (Fig. 8.1).

Treatment decision is not always possible based on a single radiograph, hence a radiograph of the antimere is frequently taken for comparison. The degree of root development of the affected tooth and the amount of dentin apposition along the canal should be compared with those of the contra lateral tooth (Fig. 8.1). It is Important to remember that the root canals of permanent teeth are wider in the bucco-lingual plane than the mesio-distal. Therefore it is difficult to determine the extent of apical closure in a regular radiograph showing only the mesio-distal plane.

In the anterior region, radiographs of each central incisor should be obtained separately from a distal angulation to prevent overlapping of the periodontal ligament of the central incisor over the lateral incisor. Performing radiography in this manner is often important in teeth after traumatic injuries (Fig. 8.2b) [1]. Lateral external inflammatory root resorption is a common finding in necrotic young teeth after trauma. External replacement root resorption can also be seen after traumatic injuries.

In recent years the use of Cone Beam Computed Tomography (CBCT) in endodontics has significantly increased. CBCT is a technique that produces undistorted three-dimensional digital imaging of the teeth and their surrounding tissues at reduced cost and less radiation for the patient than traditional CT scans.

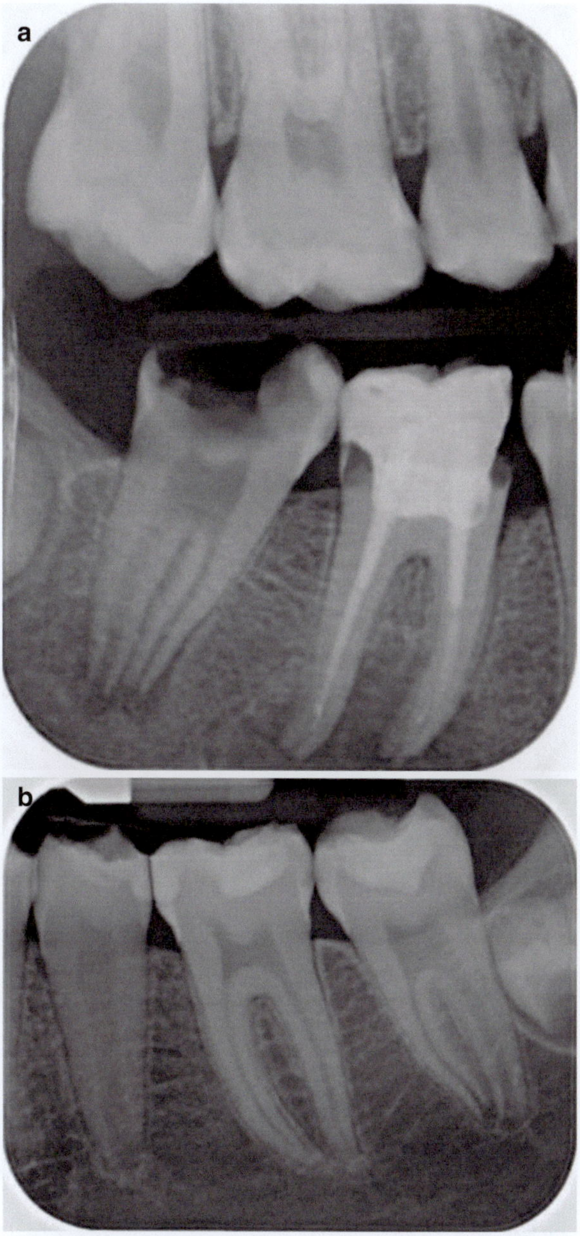

Fig. 8.1 (**a**) Vertical bite wing also used as a periapical radiograph can be used in order to demonstrate information provided by both types of radiographs. Deep carious and periapical radiolucency is observed in the mandibular permanent second molar. (**b**) Periapical radiograph of the contra lateral tooth showing normal apical papilla (Courtesy Dr. M. Raginsky)

The American Association of Endodontics (AAE) and the American Academy of Oral and Maxillofacial Radiology (AAOMR) states that the use of CBCT is justified in cases in which the benefits to the patient outweigh the potential risks of exposure to X-rays, especially in the case of children or young adults. CBCT should only be used when the question for which imaging is required cannot be

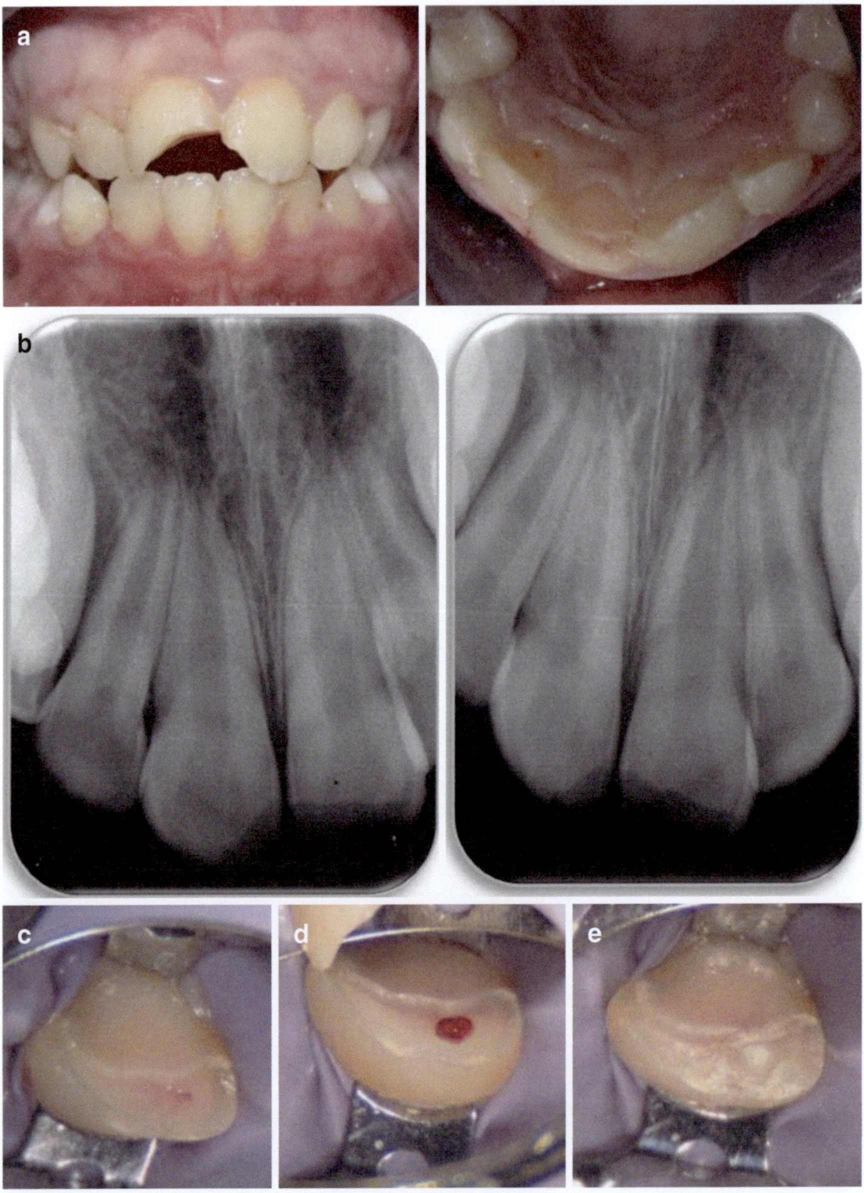

Fig. 8.2 (**a**) 9½ years old girl 4 days post complicated crown fracture in the right maxillary permanent central incisor. (**b**) Radiographs of the maxillary central incisors. Immature roots with open apices and wide root canals can be seen. (**c**) The right maxillary central incisor after cleaning and disinfection with sodium hypochlorite solution. A small pulp exposure is seen. (**d**) Partial pulpotomy. (**e**) White MTA (ProRoot, Dentsply, Tulsa, OK, USA) as pulp capping material. (**f**) Glass Ionomer (Fuji IX, GC, Leuven, Belgium) placed on top of the MTA. (**g**) Two year follow-up. Grey discoloration caused by the white MTA is seen in the crown. Continuous root formation and apical closure is evident in the radiograph (Courtesy Dr. E. Nuni)

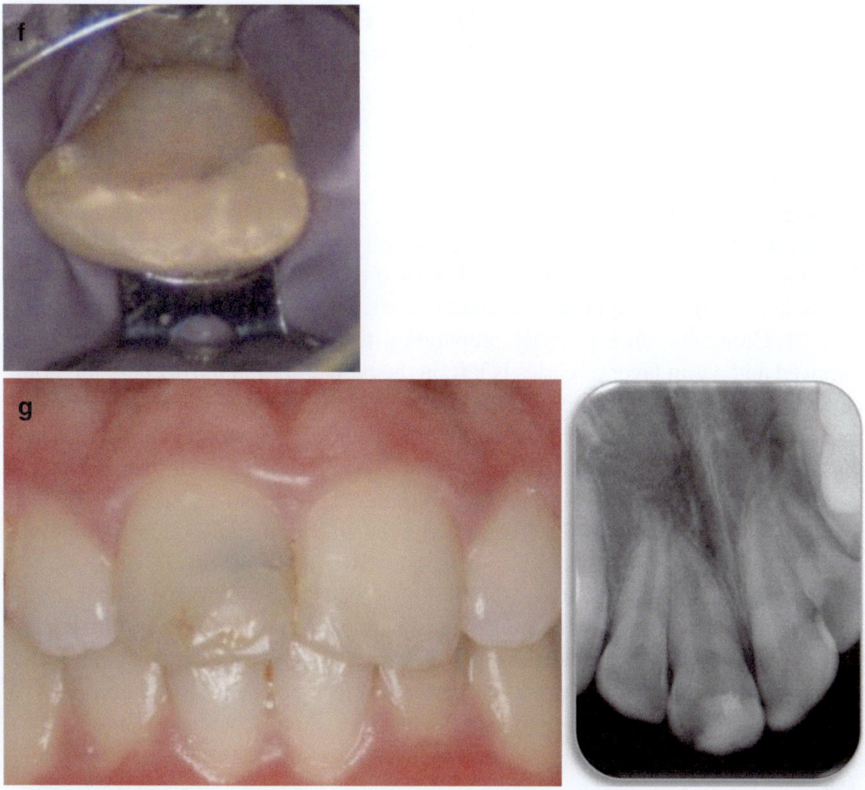

Fig. 8.2 (continued)

answered adequately by lower dose conventional dental radiography or alternate imaging modalities [12].

8.2.4 Direct Pulp Evaluation

In some instances, during the clinical treatment, a final diagnosis can only be reached by direct visualization of the pulp tissue. The appearance of the pulp tissue and the quality (color) and the amount of bleeding from a direct exposure of the pulp must be assessed; profuse or deep purple colored bleeding, or pus exudate indicates irreversible pulpitis. Based on these observations, the treatment plan may be confirmed or changed [1].

The different procedures of vital pulp therapy for *immature permanent teeth* have much in common with those of primary teeth and include indirect and direct pulp capping, partial pulpotomy, cervical pulpotomy and apexogenesis (see Chaps. 4 and 5). As mentioned, in young permanent teeth all the effort is made to preserve total or partial vitality of the pulp. Treatment procedures for *nonvital immature* permanent teeth will be presented further in this chapter.

8.3 Vital Pulp Therapy for Normal Pulp or Reversible Pulpitis *Without Pulp Exposure*

8.3.1 Indirect Pulp Treatment (IPT)

Caries excavation and indirect pulp treatment (IPT) for immature permanent teeth is similar to that of primary teeth (see Chap. 4). The main objective of indirect pulp treatment is to maintain the vitality of teeth with deep caries and reversible pulpitis, that otherwise might need endodontic therapy if the decay was completely removed. The indication for IPT should be limited to teeth without signs of irreversible pulpitis [13]. Clinically, during cavity preparation the demineralized carious tissue is removed and a thin layer of caries is left on the pulpal floor at the deepest site of the cavity to avoid pulp exposure. The carious tissue is then covered with a biocompatible material. The materials most commonly used in IPT are calcium hydroxide, glass ionomer and Mineral Trioxide Aggregate (MTA). The tooth then is restored with a material that seals the tooth from microleakage.

Two clinical procedures have been described in the literature: one appointment caries excavation and a step-wise technique (two appointments) (see Chap. 4). Research available is inconclusive on which approach is the most successful over time [14, 15]. Several studies have demonstrated a high percentage of success utilizing IPT *both in permanent and primary teeth* [15–17]. Rickets et al. have demonstrates that in symptomless, vital, carious primary or permanent teeth, stepwise and partial excavation reduced the risk of pulp exposure. Therefore these techniques show clinical advantage over complete caries removal in the management of dentinal caries [16].

8.4 Vital Pulp Therapy for Normal Pulp or Reversible Pulpitis *With Pulp Exposure*

8.4.1 Direct Pulp Capping

Direct pulp capping may be performed when a *small exposure* of the pulp is encountered during cavity preparation in teeth with a normal pulp or reversible pulpitis, or following a recently sustained traumatic injury [18]. The aim of this treatment is to maintain pulp vitality by forming a calcified barrier (reparative dentin) to wall off the exposure. It should be kept in mind that, in teeth affected by caries, there is an inflammatory response of the pulp to bacteria or bacterial products [19, 20].

Direct pulp capping should be performed immediately after the exposure to prevent contamination of the pulp. As the extent of the inflammatory process in the pulp cannot be accurately assessed by clinical tests, the diagnosis of reversible (treatable) pulpitis may be sometimes incorrect. In some teeth affected by deep caries, pulp inflammation might have reached the stage of irreversible pulpitis without showing clinical signs.

The characteristics of the pulp capping material are of significant importance: it should ideally be biocompatible, non-resorbable, capable of establishing and maintaining a good seal to prevent bacterial contamination, and capable of promoting pulp repair and dentin bridge formation. Ideally the dentin bridge formed after direct pulp capping should be without tunnel defects that could allow the penetration of bacteria into the pulp at a later stage [1].

Mineral trioxide aggregate (MTA) and calcium hydroxide are the most frequently recommended capping materials. The mechanism of action of the two materials in vital pulp treatment are similar, as the main soluble component of MTA is calcium hydroxide [21]. Calcium hydroxide dissolves in an aqueous environment into calcium and hydroxyl ions creating a high pH in the close environment (~12). This alkaline pH is responsible for the antibacterial activity of these materials [22]. The initial effect of calcium hydroxide applied to an exposed pulp tissue is the development of a superficial necrosis as a result of the high pH. This necrosis causes low-grade irritation to the tissue and stimulates the pulp to defense and repair. Contrary to calcium hydroxide, MTA causes mild inflammatory and necrotic changes in the subjacent pulp. Thus it is less caustic than the traditional calcium hydroxide preparations [23]. Calcium ions are released from the capping material, forming inorganic precipitations that have been associated with the mechanism controlling cytological and functional changes in the interacting pulpal cells [24].

The high pH and low solubility of calcium hydroxide prolongs its antibacterial effect. However, being water soluble, it might dissolve under leaky restorations and be washed out, leaving an empty space under the filling material. Hard-setting calcium hydroxide cements can induce dentin bridge formation, but they do not provide an effective long-term seal against bacteria or their by-products [1].

Recent studies suggest that the mechanisms by which calcium hydroxide or MTA stimulate the wound healing process is related to the solubilizing effect of calcium hydroxide on the dentin matrix component. Growth factors and other bioactive molecules, sequestered within the dentin matrix during dentinogenesis (e.g., TGF-βs) may be released by the action of calcium hydroxide and mediate the changes in cell behavior observed during reparative dentinogenesis [4, 25].

MTA presents some advantages over calcium hydroxide as the material of choice for direct pulp capping. It is a hard setting biocompatible material with an antibacterial effect that provides a biologically active substrate for cell attachment. These features make this material effective in preventing microleakage, improving the treatment outcome. As previously mentioned, MTA stimulates reparative dentin formation with negligible pulpal necrosis and minimal inflammatory reaction in the exposed pulp [23]. Tziafas demonstrated that after direct pulp capping with MTA in dogs the underlying pulp tissue was consistently normal, and only at a later stage some hemorrhage in the pulp core was observed. The beginning of a hard tissue barrier was observed after 2 weeks, and reparative dentinogenesis was disclosed after 3 weeks, associated with a firm fibrodentin matrix [26]. It was also demonstrated that, compared with calcium hydroxide, MTA consistently induces the formation of dentin bridge at a greater rate with a superior structural integrity. Therefore, MTA appears to be more effective than calcium hydroxide for maintaining long-term pulp vitality after direct pulp capping [23].

However, MTA presents a major drawback by staining tooth material, both in the grey and white versions [27, 28] (Fig. 8.2e,g). Hence, its use in vital pulp therapy procedures (pulp capping, pulpotomy) is not recommended in teeth where there is an esthetic concern. In these teeth alternatives to MTA (such as calcium hydroxide) should be considered.

Biodentine™ (Septodont, Allington Maidstone, Kent ME16 OJZ UK) is a new generation calcium silicate based material (as MTA) which is described by the manufacturer as bioactive and biocompatible dentin substitute. It was introduced to the dental market in 2009 and its properties have been described as similar to MTA. Its main advantage over MTA is its short setting time, ~10 min, which enables the completion of some clinical procedures in one visit vs. two. It also appears that Biodentine does not cause tooth discoloration, but further studies are needed in this matter [29, 30].

Direct pulp capping should always be followed by an immediate and definitive restoration.

8.4.1.1 Direct Pulp Capping Technique

The tooth should be isolated with a rubber dam and disinfected with sodium hypochlorite (NaOCl) solution. During cavity preparation with high speed burs under constant water spray and caries removal with low speed burs, the cavity should be rinsed with sodium hypochlorite from time to time to decrease the bacterial load. No further pulpal tissue is removed except that occurring with the caries removal. Pulpal hemorrhage is controlled by copious irrigation with NaOCl solution [31]. The solution is refreshed every 3–4 min and may be left in contact with the exposed pulp tissue for about 10 min. NaOCl disinfects the cavity and removes the blood clot from the pulp exposure site. Care should be taken to remove the blood clot prior to placement of the dressing material over the exposed pulp, as its presence may compromise the treatment outcome. It has been demonstrated that leaving the blood clot may result in the formation of dystrophic calcifications and internal resorption. It may also interfere with dentin bridge formation and serve as a substrate for bacteria in leaky restorations [32]. NaOCl appears to have no adverse effect on pulpal healing and dentin bridge formation [31].

If the bleeding cannot be controlled within 10 min, it appears that pulp inflammation is more extensive and has progressed deeper into the tissue. Therefore, a tooth initially scheduled for a direct pulp cap may be a better candidate for a pulpotomy [33]. After hemorrhage control, MTA (or calcium hydroxide) should be prepared according to the manufacturer's instructions and placed directly over the exposed pulp tissue (1.5–2 mm thick). The material should then be covered with a glass ionomer liner followed by a permanent restoration with an excellent sealing ability.

8.4.2 Pulpotomy

Although the use of direct pulp capping and pulpotomy in cariously exposed pulps of mature teeth remains a controversial issue in Endodontics, these procedures are universally accepted in young immature permanent teeth. The pulpotomy procedure involves removing pulp tissue that has inflammatory or degenerative changes, leaving intact the remaining clinically appearing healthy tissue, which is then covered with a pulp-capping agent to promote healing at the amputation site. The only difference between pulpotomy and pulp capping is that in pulpotomy additional tissue is removed from the exposed pulp. Traditionally, pulpotomy implied the removal of the entire coronal pulp up to the cervical area. Today the depth of tissue removal is based on clinical judgment: only tissue with profuse bleeding, judged to be inflamed or infected, should be removed, as the capping material should be placed on healthy tissue [1].

Although many materials and drugs have been used as capping agents after pulpotomy, MTA seems to be the treatment of choice to stimulate dentin bridge formation in young permanent teeth with exposed pulps [23]. In aesthetic areas MTA is not recommended because of its discoloration effect. Calcium hydroxide may be used as its outcomes are similar in some studies [34, 35]. Aguilar reported that partial pulpotomy and full (cervical) pulpotomy provide a more predictable outcome than direct pulp capping in teeth with carious exposure [33].

8.4.2.1 Partial (Cvek) Pulpotomy Technique

Partial pulpotomy was first presented by Cvek as a treatment modality for traumatic pulp exposures after complicated crown fracture [36]. Cvek and his collogues have shown that in untreated traumatic pulp exposures the pulp inflammatory reaction is usually proliferative (hyperplasia), and the inflammation extends not more than 2 mm into the pulp tissue even after 7 days. Therefore they recommended that not more than 2 mm of the pulp beneath the exposure needs to be removed in these cases (Fig. 8.2) [37].

The tooth should be isolated with a rubber dam and disinfected with NaOCl solution. In traumatically exposed pulps, only tissue judged to be inflamed should be removed (~2 mm). In teeth with carious exposure, it might be necessary to remove tissue to a greater depth in order to reach non-inflamed pulp. Care should be taken to remove all the tissue coronal to the amputation site to prevent continuation of bleeding, contamination, and discoloration of the tooth. Cutting of the tissue with an abrasive high speed diamond bur with water cooling, has been shown to be the least damaging to the underlying tissue [38].

After pulp amputation, the preparation is thoroughly washed with NaOCl to disinfect and control hemorrhage. If hemorrhage persists, amputation should be performed at a more apical level [33]. Once hemorrhage has been controlled, a dressing of MTA (or calcium hydroxide in aesthetic area) is gently placed over the amputation site. Care should be taken not to push the material into the pulp [39]. The MTA should be covered with a glass ionomer liner and a permanent restoration should be placed. If the pulpotomy is successful, a tertiary dentin bridge will be formed, and occasionally pulp obliteration may occur (Fig. 8.2) [1].

8.4.2.2 Cervical (full) Pulpotomy

Cervical pulpotomy in *mature teeth* is performed only when irreversible pulpitis is diagnosed, and it should be considered as an emergency treatment. In these teeth, root canal treatment will follow at the next appointment.

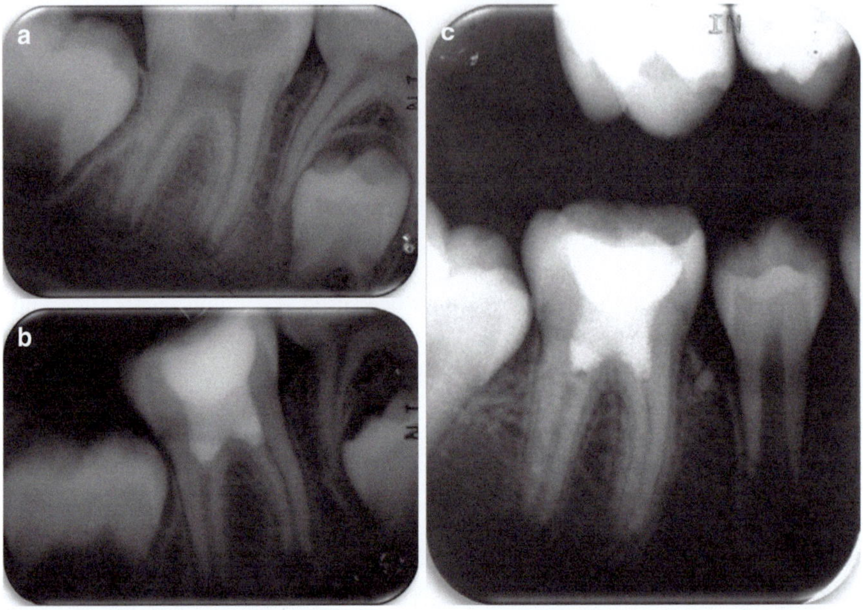

Fig. 8.3 (**a**) 9 years old girl. First right lower permanent molar with a very deep caries lesion. The tooth is asymptomatic and respond with mild pain to cold test. Radiographically an immature roots with very open apices are observed. (**b**) After cervical pulpotomy. White MTA (ProRoot®, Dentsply, Tulsa, OK, USA) is seen in the canal orifices covered with a layer of GI. The crown was restored with composite. (**c**) 2 years follow-up. Continuous root maturation is evident with no signs of apical pathosis (Courtesy Dr. E. Nuni)

In immature permanent teeth, cervical pulpotomy is performed to allow maturation of the root (Fig. 8.3). This procedure is performed in teeth in which it is assumed that healthy pulp tissue, with a potential to produce a dentin bridge and complete the formation of the root, still remains in the root canal [1].

The technique for cervical pulpotomy is similar to that for partial pulpotomy except for the level of pulp tissue amputation. In cervical pulpotomy the entire coronal pulp is carefully amputated using a sharp excavator or a slow-speed large round bur to the level of the canal orifice. MTA (or calcium hydroxide) is used as dressing material in order to maintain pulp vitality and function. It is of utmost importance to perform a permanent restoration as soon as possible to prevent bacterial leakage and ensure the success of the treatment (Fig. 8.3b).

Cervical pulpotomy is frequently performed in teeth in which the histopathologic status of the pulp stumps is not clear. If the symptoms continue and pulpectomy is needed the MTA may be removed gently using an ultrasonic instrument and an operative microscope [1].

Follow-up After Vital Pulp Therapy

Clinical and radiographic follow-up of these teeth is essential because pulp necrosis, canal obliteration and root resorption are possible sequelae of vital pulp therapy.

No adverse clinical signs or symptoms of sensitivity, pain, or swelling should be present. Radiographically, no signs of internal or external resorption nor periapical radiolucency should be found. The roots should show continued normal development and maturogenesis in teeth with incompletely formed roots.

In some cases continuous calcification of the root canals is noticed after vital pulp therapy. There is a controversy weather root canal treatment is indicated after achieving root maturation, before obliteration of the root canal space occurs that will prevent performing root canal treatment in the future. Routine prophylactic endodontic treatment is contraindicated because of the low percentage of pulp necrosis [40, 41]. Root canal treatment can be considered in posterior teeth, where apicectomy is difficult to perform in cases of treatment failure, especially in children.

8.4.3 Apexogenesis

Apexogenesis is indicated in immature permanent teeth when the inflammation of the pulp tissue is considered to be so deep, that only part of the tissue inside the root canal is presumed to be vital and healthy. This procedure allows continued physiologic development and maturation of the root apex apical to the dressing material. The root formed may be irregular but nevertheless provides additional support for the tooth. Apexogenesis can be clinically regarded as a very deep pulpotomy therefore, the technique is similar. The use of the operative microscope is recommended in order to execute this meticulous procedure correctly. MTA or calcium hydroxide is placed over the pulp stump after hemostasis control with NaOCl (Fig. 8.4).

It is difficult to determine the pulp status deep in the root canal or to predict the formation of a calcified barrier and continued root development. Clinical and radiographic follow-up is mandatory, and if signs and/or symptoms of pathology appear, apexification or pulp regenerative procedure should follow. The use of MTA as a dressing material should be carefully considered because of the difficulty in removing the material from deep inside the root canal [1].

8.5 Nonvital Pulp Treatment for Immature Teeth

8.5.1 Apexification

Apexification is a method of treatment for immature permanent teeth in which root growth and development ceased due to pulp necrosis. Its purpose is to induce root end closure by forming a calcified barrier with no canal wall thickening nor continuous root lengthening, as the Hertwig's epithelial root sheath (HERS) is absent. As previously mentioned, diagnosing pulp necrosis in immature teeth can be challenging due to confounding factors such as the normal radiographic radiolucency visible at the root end in these teeth and the unreliability of sensibility tests (Fig. 8.1b).

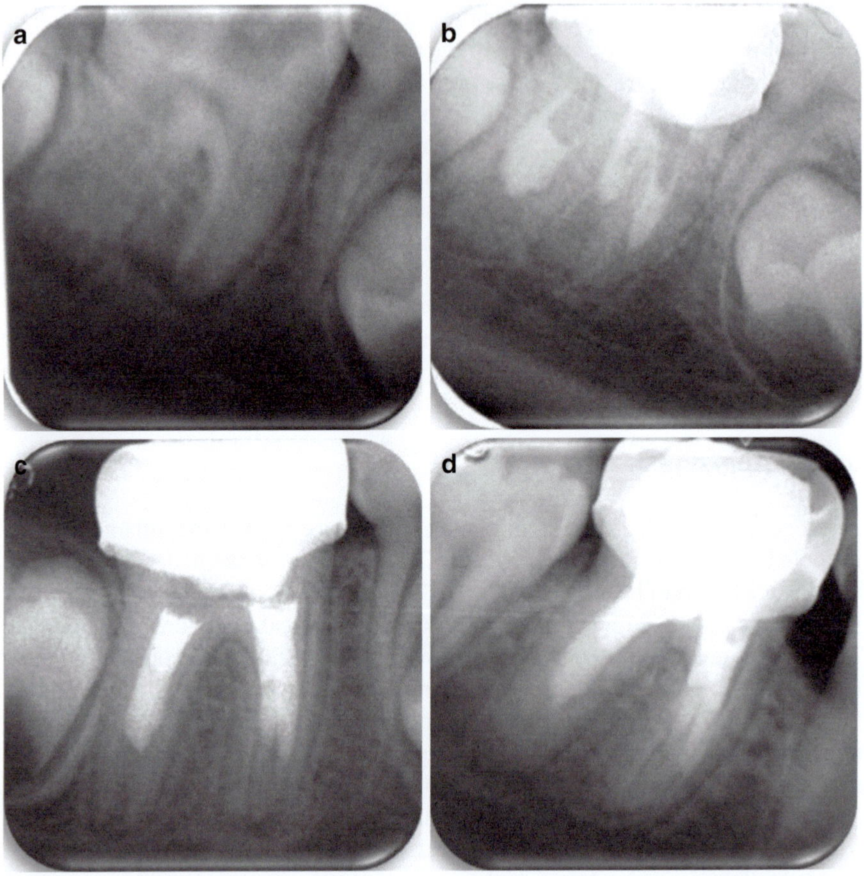

Fig. 8.4 (**a**) 7 years old boy. First right lower permanent molar with a very deep caries lesion. Radiographically an immature root with very wide blunderbuss shaped open apices are observed. (**b**) After removal of pulp tissue from the pulp chamber and the coronal part of the canals a tissue judged to be non-inflamed was seen with the help of the operative microscope. White MTA (ProRoot®, Detsply, Tulsa, OK, USA) was placed on the healthy tissue. (Metal crown was placed in order to achieve isolation from the oral cavity). (**c**) On the next visit the MTA was found to be hard and gutta-percha and sealer were used to obdurate the coronal part of the canals. (**d**) 4 years follow-up. Complete development of the apical part of the roots is seen with no evidence of periapical pathosis (Courtesy Dr. E. Nuni)

Apexification should only be performed when the diagnosis of pulp necrosis is certain. It can be achieved in two ways: the traditional long term procedure using calcium hydroxide dressing to stimulate the formation of a biologic hard tissue barrier, and the more recently short term procedure, creating an artificial apical plug with MTA. Apexification is most often performed in anterior teeth that lost vitality due to a traumatic injury or a deep carious lesion, and in teeth with anatomic variations such as *dens invaginatus* with an immature root.

The open apex of immature teeth may present a few morphological variations. It can be divergent with flaring apical foramen (blunderbuss apex), parallel, or convergent. The exact morphology is difficult to determine because of the two-dimensional

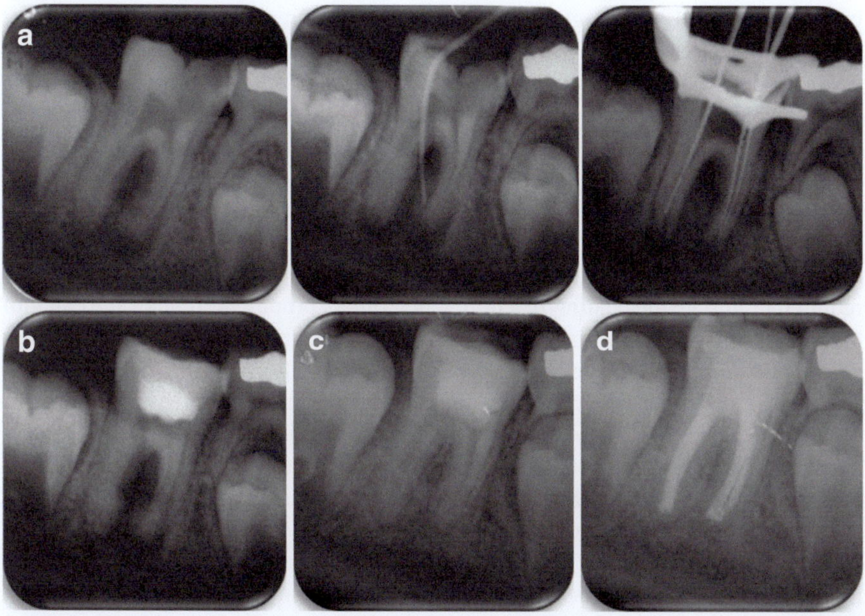

Fig. 8.5 (**a**) 8½ years old girl. First right lower permanent molar with a very deep caries lesion and buccal sinus tract. Radiographically a large radiolucent lesion around the roots and the bifurcation is seen. Tracing radiograph with gutta-percha master cone leads to this area. (**b**) Radiographic appearance after packing of the canals with thick calcium hydroxide paste in the second visit. The roots look obliterated because the radio-opacity of thick calcium hydroxide paste resembles that of dentin. (**c**) Six months after calcium hydroxide packing. The radiolucent area is almost completely resolved and a calcified barrier is seen in the apical area of the canals. (**d**) Final radiograph (2 months after **c**) showing obturation of the root canals with gutta-percha and sealer (Courtesy Dr. E. Nuni)

image obtained by dental radiographs. In all of these variations endodontic treatment cannot be performed, as it is difficult, if not impossible, to achieve an apical seal that will prevent extrusion of the filling material.

Follow up should be performed in order to ensure the absence of adverse post-treatment clinical symptoms and/or radiographic signs of pathology. When the procedure is carried out successfully in teeth with radiographic signs of rarifying osteitis, healing of the bone will be observed gradually, the tooth will continue to erupt and the alveolar bone will continue to grow in conjunction with the adjacent teeth.

Publications in the last decade present an alternative treatment to apexification in the form of pulp regenerative therapy even in cases of infected necrotic immature teeth. This will be discussed further in this chapter.

8.5.1.1 Long Term Apexification with Calcium Hydroxide

Apexification is traditionally performed using a calcium hydroxide dressing (Fig. 8.5) [42]. It is a predictable procedure, and an apical barrier will be formed in 74–100 % of cases [43]. This procedure demands multiple visits and requires patient and parent compliance, as it could take a year or more to achieve a complete apical barrier that would allow a gutta-percha root canal filling. It is unclear whether the stage of root development at the beginning of the treatment or the presence of a pre-treatment infection affect the time required for barrier formation [44].

Calcium hydroxide assists in the debridement of the root canal, as it increases the dissolution of necrotic tissue when used alone or in combination with NaOCl [45]. The high pH and low solubility of calcium hydroxide keeps its antimicrobial effect in the root canal for a long period of time [46, 47]. Disagreement still exists as to whether or how often the calcium hydroxide dressing should be changed. Some investigators support a single application of the material and claim that it is only required to initiate the healing reaction, while others propose to replace the calcium hydroxide only when symptoms develop or if the material appears to have been washed out of the canal when viewed radiographically [44].

The calcified barrier is formed by cells originating from the adjacent connective tissue, but the mechanism of action of calcium hydroxide in induction of an apical barrier remains controversial. The calcified barrier, although appearing clinically and radiographically complete, is histologically porous and may be composed of cementum, dentin, bone or osteodentin [44].

The most severe complication of calcium hydroxide apexification is cervical root fracture [3]. Studies have shown that long-term dressing that would expose root dentin to calcium hydroxide for periods exceeding one month results in structural changes in the dentin, with higher susceptibility to root fracture [48, 49].

Calcium Hydroxide Apexification Technique

Rubber dam isolation is mandatory. The coronal access should be wide enough to include the pulp horns to prevent future contamination and discoloration (Fig. 8.5). In anterior teeth, Gates-Glidden drills can be used to remove the palatal eminence in the cervical portion of the root canal, facilitating cleaning of all aspects of the canal. The length of the root canal should be determined radiographically with a large gutta percha point (Fig. 8.6a) or endodontic files (Fig. 8.5a), as electronic apex locator is not reliable in teeth with open apices. Inserting a large size paper point to the point of bleeding may also assist in length determination. The working length should be approximately 1 mm short of the radiographic root end [1].

Debridement of the root canal, is mainly achieved by irrigation with NaOCl solution utilizing its excellent tissue-dissolving properties and its antimicrobial efficacy [50]. The irrigation should be done carefully without pressure, verifying that the needle is loose inside the root canal and short of the working length. Passive ultrasonic irrigation with NaOCl solution is recommended in order to facilitate disinfection and debris removal from these wide canals [51]. Minimal or no instrumentation is advised to prevent damage to the thin dentin walls. A calcium hydroxide dressing in a creamy consistency can then be applied into the canal space with a Lentulo spiral, specially designed syringes or files.

A second visit is scheduled 2–4 weeks later. Its aim is to complete the debridement and remove the tissue remnants denaturized by the calcium hydroxide dressing that could not be removed mechanically in the first appointment and to further disinfect the canal. After disinfection a thick paste of calcium hydroxide is packed

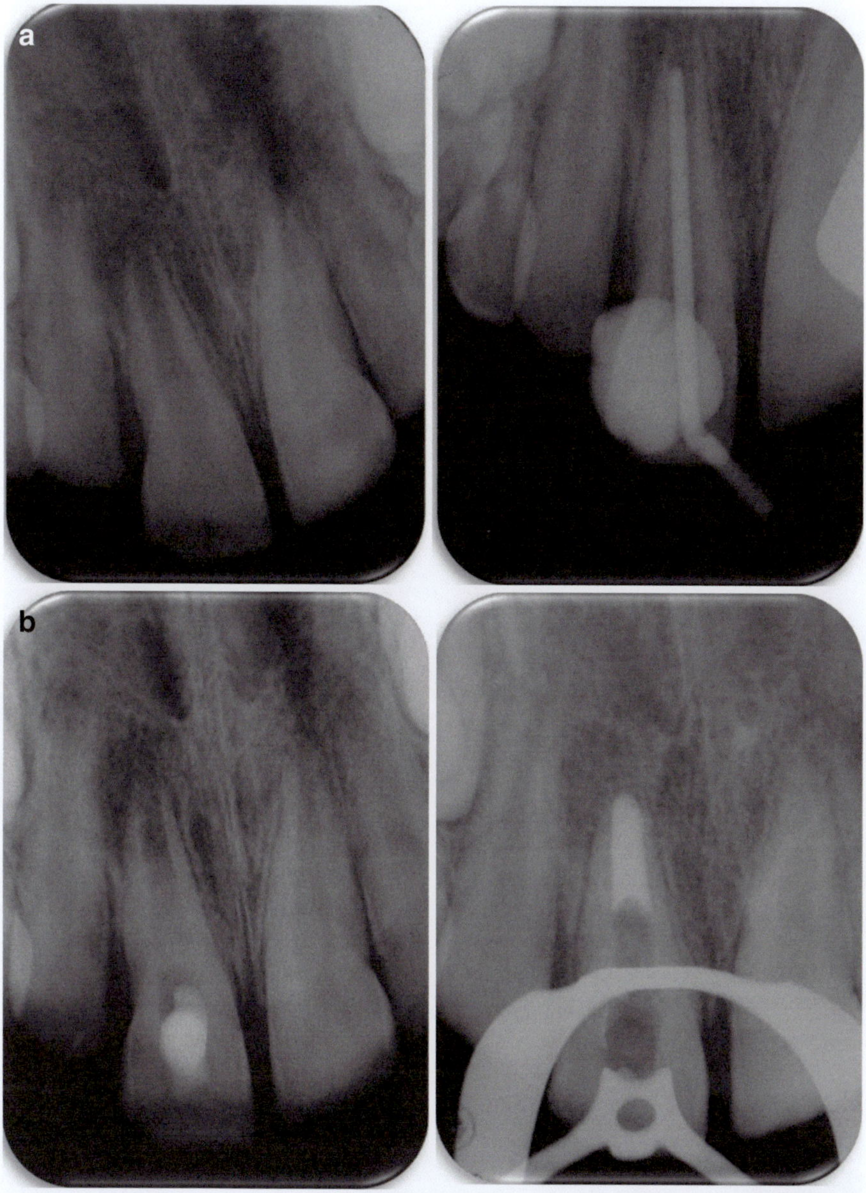

Fig. 8.6 (**a**, *left*) 10 years old boy 10 months post dental trauma (11- subluxation + uncomplicated crown fracture). The upper right central incisor presents no clinical symptoms with negative respond to cold test. Radiographically an immature root with open apex and radiolucent periapical lesion is observed. (**a**, *right*) Working length radiograph with gutta percha point. (**b**, *left*) One month after debridement and dressing with creamy calcium hydroxide paste. (**b**, *right*) MTA apical plague placement. (**c**, *left*) Set white MTA apical plague (1 month after its placement). (**c**, *right*) Permanent restoration with bonding of glass fibers in light curing resin matrix (everStick™, GC Corporation, Tokyo, Japan) is performed in direct contact with the set MTA plague. (**d**) 2 years follow up. Complete resolution of the apical radiolucency is evident (Courtesy Dr. E. Nuni)

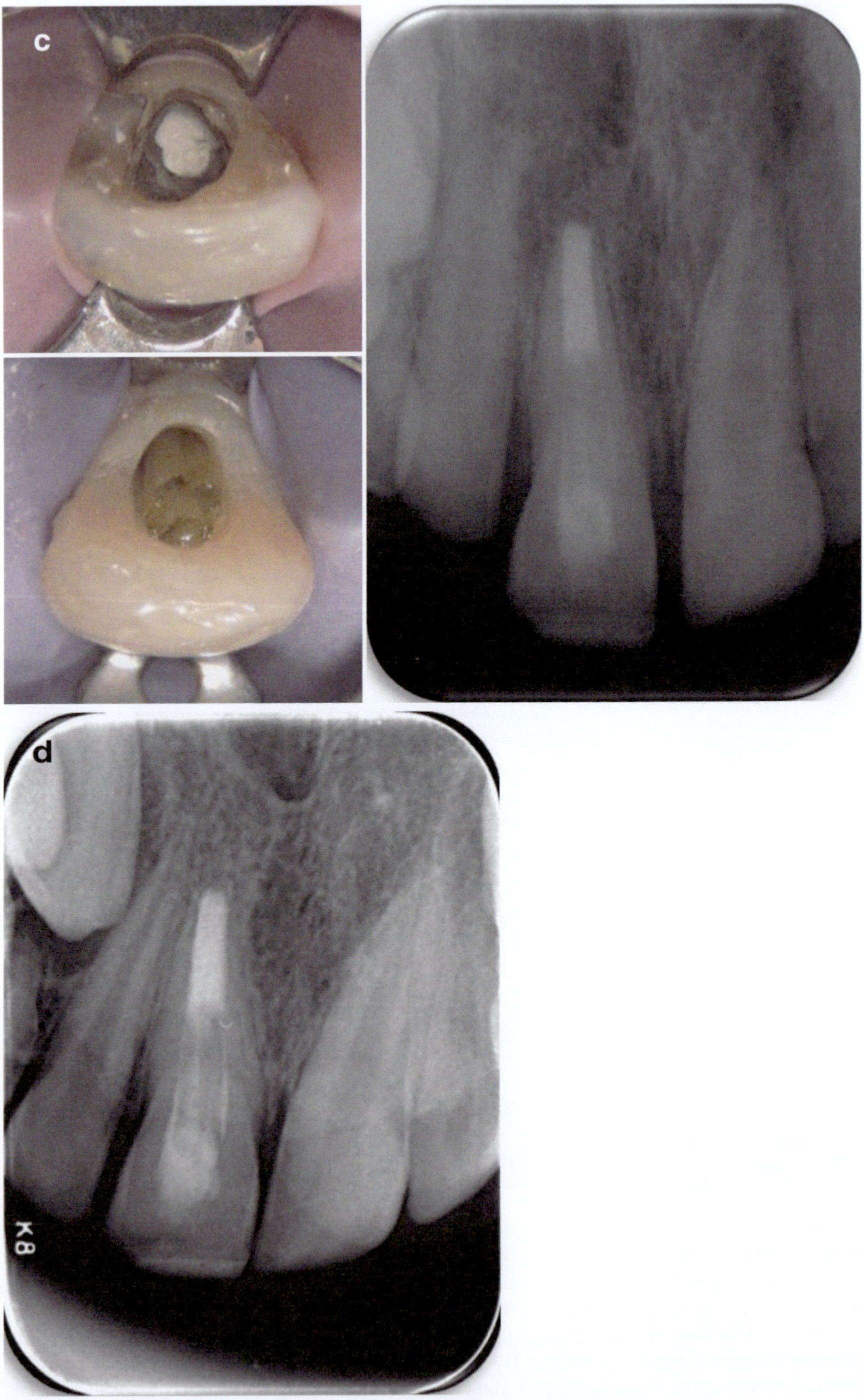

Fig. 8.6 (continued)

in the root canal using endodontic pluggers (Fig. 8.5b) [52]. The dressing is packed to a level apical to the cemento-enamel junction (CEJ) in order to reduce dentin weakening in this fracture sensitive area. The coronal access should be restored with a filling that provide a long term coronal seal.

The tooth should be monitored clinically and radiographically at 3-months intervals to examine the formation of an apical hard tissue barrier and ensure the absence of pathologies. If a calcified barrier is not evident and the calcium hydroxide has been washed out, its replacement is usually indicated. When a calcified barrier can be seen on the radiograph, the tooth is reopened and the calcium hydroxide is removed by copious irrigation. The apical area should be gently examined using a gutta percha point and/or through the operative microscope in order to determine the completeness of the apical barrier. If the barrier is incomplete, the apexification procedure is reestablished until a complete barrier is formed [1].

After the formation of a complete apical barrier the canal is obturated with a permanent root canal filling material (e.g., thermoplasticized gutta-percha) and sealer (Fig. 8.5d). When a calcified barrier is formed coronal to the apex, it should not be perforated in order to fill the canal to the apical end; the tissue forming the apical barrier should be regarded as healthy tissue and root canal filling should be placed up to this point.

Immature teeth with thin dentin walls, especially after calcium hydroxide apexification, are at high risk of fracture. The stage of root development seems to be a key factor [3, 49]. In order to reduce this risk a permanent restoration with an intra-canal placement of bonded composite resin is recommended (Fig. 8.6c, *right*) [53].

8.5.1.2 Short Term Apexification With MTA (One Visit Apexification)

The use of MTA as an artificial apical plug instead of the long traditional apexification with calcium hydroxide is widespread for more than a decade (Fig. 8.6). Its main advantage lies in reducing the time needed for completion of the root canal treatment and the restoration of the tooth. An artificial apical barrier is placed in one visit while the whole treatment is completed in just few frequent visits [54]. Characteristics such as low solubility, excellent sealability, biocompatibility, release of calcium hydroxide, high pH and radiopacity are responsible for the preferable clinical results and popularity of MTA as an apical plug material [55].

Disinfection of the root canal is achieved in the first visit as described in the long term apexification with calcium hydroxide. At the second visit MTA can be placed in the apical portion of the immature root and will act as an apical plug after setting. It is difficult to remove the MTA from within the canal after it sets (even with the use of the operative microscope and advanced ultrasonic instruments) [27] and in case of treatment failure apical surgery may be indicated. Therefore complete debridement and disinfection of the root canal and of the dentin walls is mandatory.

One visit apexification presents a number of advantages: shortens treatment time, improves patient compliance, reduces cost and clinical time, the dentin will not lose its physical properties and rapid placement of a bonded restoration within the root canal is possible, thus minimizing the likelihood of root fracture.

MTA Apexification Technique

Disinfection of the root canal is achieved as described in the first visit of the long term apexification. Calcium hydroxide dressing is also indicated in order to raise the low pH of the inflamed periapical tissue before the MTA placement. Lee et al. have demonstrated that an acidic environment has an adverse effect on the setting and micro hardness of MTA [56].

In the second visit, after rubber dam placement, the canal is irrigated and dried. After mixing according to the manufacturer's instructions a plug of MTA is compacted into the apical 4–5 mm of the canal, about 1 mm short of the radiographic apex (Fig. 8.6b, *right*). Placement of MTA in the apical part is more complicated than the use of calcium hydroxide. The material is introduced into the apical area using special carriers or endodontic pluggers and compacted using hand condensation with indirect ultrasonic activation [57]. Placement of a resorbable material at the root end (e.g., calcium sulfate, CollaCote™, Zimmer Dental, Carlsbad, CA, USA) against which the MTA can be compacted keeping it within the confines of the canal space has been suggested but does not seem necessary [58, 59]. Proper placement of the material is verified by a radiograph (Fig. 8.6b, *right*). A wet cotton pellet or paper point is placed over the MTA providing moisture for its setting and the tooth is sealed with a temporary filling.

After a few days the tooth is reentered and the hardness of the MTA is examined with an endodontic instrument. In case that the MTA is not set, its placement should be repeated the same way described. After setting, the root canal filling can be completed using thermoplasticized gutta-percha and sealer. The tooth is then permanently restored with a bonded composite resin extending into the canal space in an attempt to strengthen the root [53]. In short roots the composite resin can be placed in direct contact with the MTA plug (Fig. 8.6c, *right*).

Using a new generation calcium silicate based material (e.g., Biodentine™ Allington Maidstone, Kent ME16 OJZ UK) can shorten the treatment period even further. The short setting time of this material (~10 min) will allow the placement of a permanent root filling and tooth restoration at the same visit of the apical plug placement.

8.5.2 Pulp Revascularization and Regeneration

The traditionally recommended clinical treatment for immature nonvital/infected teeth with wide open apices is apexification as described above. Continuous root maturation is impossible in teeth receiving apexification and the immature root left is short, weak and fracture-prone [2, 3], with a risk of increased tooth mobility due to the compromised crown-to-root ratio.

For more than a decade this paradigm has been challenged by reports in the literature (mainly case reports/series), showing that immature teeth clinically diagnosed with nonvital pulp and periradicular periodontitis or abscess, can present radiographically signs of continuous root development after a clinical procedure most commonly called revascularization [2, 60, 61]. This procedure is based on the fact that under certain conditions revascularization of traumatized or auto-transplanted teeth with open apices is possible and sometimes even predictable. Studies suggests that the devitalized pulp tissue act as a scaffold into which the new vascularized tissue can grow [62–64]. It has been demonstrated that a wide apical foramen (more than 1 mm) enables better ingrowth of new tissue and a shorter extra-oral time (less than 45 min) decreases the risk of infection, improving the chance for revascularization [62, 65]. Therefore, creating similar conditions in necrotic and even infected immature teeth will allow ingrowth of new blood vessels and tissue into the pulp space. These conditions include effective disinfection of the canal, creation of a scaffold into which new tissue can grow and effective sealing of the coronal access [61].

Regeneration of functional pulpal tissue is the ideal treatment for immature necrotic permanent teeth. Murray et al. defined regenerative endodontics as "biologically based procedures designed to replace damaged structures, including dentin and root structures, as well as cells of the pulp-dentin complex" [66]. The formation of the new tissue will reproduce both the anatomy and function of the original tissue. Tissue repair however represents development of a replacement tissue, such as scar tissue, without restoration of function.

Nygaard-Ostby et al. in their classic case series were one of the first to present the concept of regenerating new pulpal tissue in the canal space. They showed ingrowth of fibrous connective tissue and cementum (repair) after evoking bleeding by over-instrumentation in human or dog root canal systems [67–69]. The exact nature of the new tissue that repopulate the canal space in the recent reports is unclear [2]. Therefore, several terms were suggested to describe the introduction of new living tissue into the canal, including; *revascularization* [61], *revitalization* [70], *regeneration* [66], *induced or guided tissue generation* [71] and *maturogenesis* [71, 72]. There is a debate between investigators as to which of these terms is most appropriate to describe the outcome of this procedure [71, 73].

A few factors are necessary for a successful endodontic regeneration. These factors include: absence of infection within the root canal space, a physical scaffold, stem cells, signaling molecules and an effective coronal seal [72, 74].

8.5.2.1 Revascularization Clinical Procedure

A variety of approaches and clinical protocols have been used for this clinical procedure. These differ in case selection, technique, materials used (irrigation, intracanal medicament and barrier), number and timing of appointments, final restoration and the treatment outcome and success [2, 75]. The AAE Regenerative Endodontics Committee publish a document (found on the AAE website) entitled "Considerations for Regenerative Procedures" [76]. It is based on the best available data at the time and is revised regularly. It is recommended as one possible source of information for clinicians to make treatment decisions, because of the rapid evolving nature of this field. The recommendations of this chapter are based on this publication.

Case Selection

Revascularization is indicated in teeth with necrotic pulp, with or without apical pathosis, and an immature apex (Fig. 8.7a). The etiology for pulp necrosis (trauma/dental anomalies/caries) does not appear to be a factor in case selection. Immature

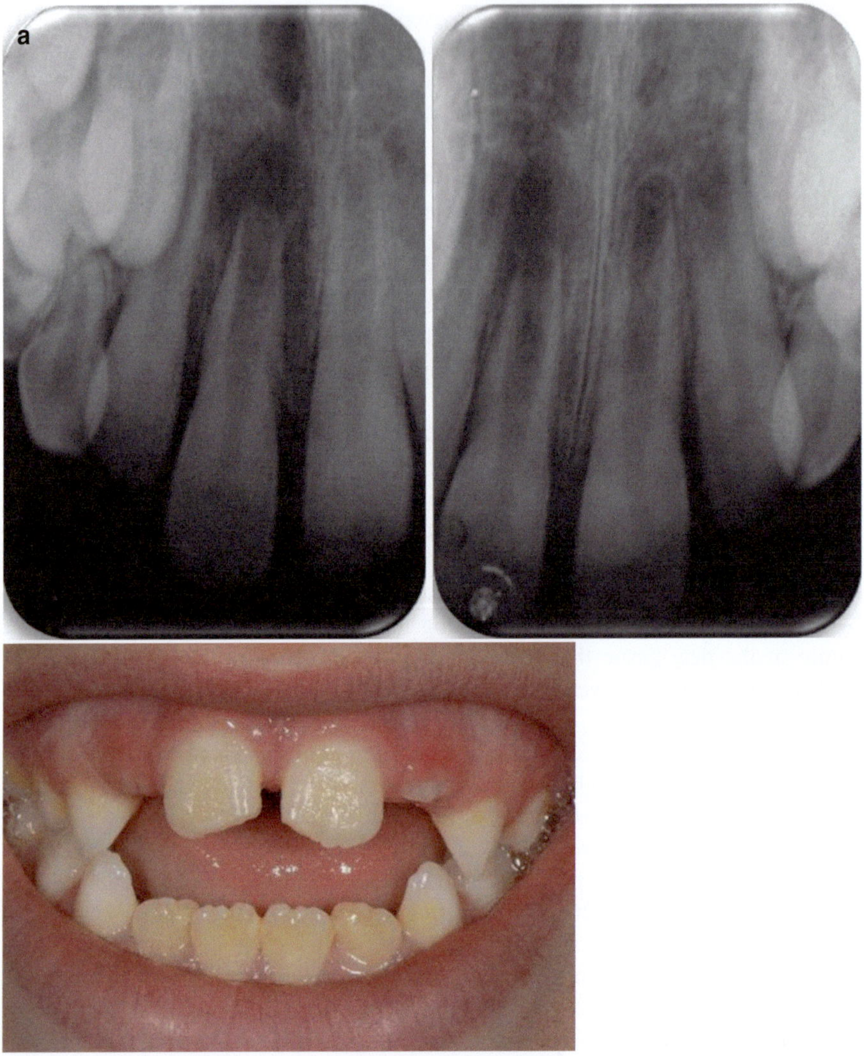

Fig. 8.7 (**a**) 7½ years old boy 4 months post dental trauma (11 + 21- uncomplicated crown fracture). The upper right central incisor presents sensitivity to percussion and negative respond to cold test. Radiographically an immature root with wide open apex and radiolucent periapical lesion is observed. (**b**) Post revascularization with triple antibiotic paste. MTA was placed over the blood clot in the root canal. (**c**) 6 months follow-up. Complete resolution of the periapical lesion & continuous PDL is evident. Thickening of the canal walls with no elongation of the root can be observed. (**d**) A 11/2 years follow-up. Greyish discoloration of the crown and continuous buildup of hard tissue along the canal walls is seen. The nature of this tissue is unclear. (**e**) 4 years follow up. Discoloration of the crown and almost complete obliteration of the canal space is observed (Courtesy Dr. E. Nuni)

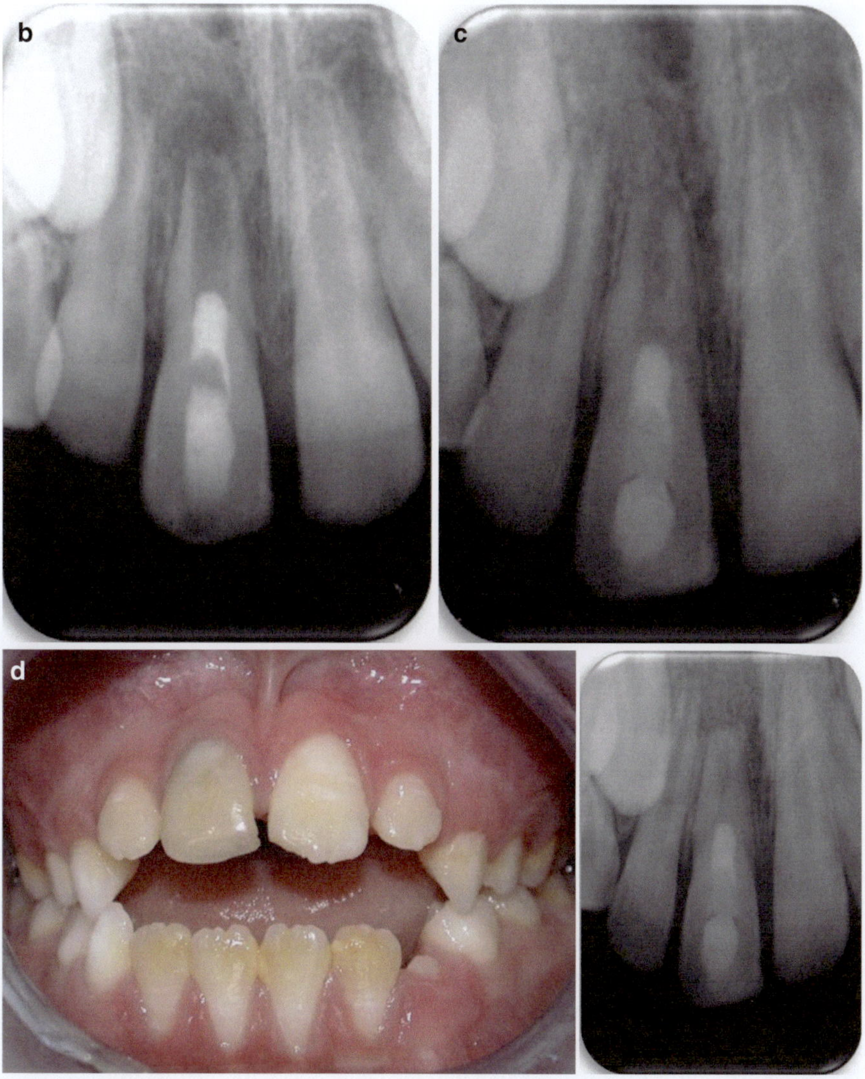

Fig. 8.7 (continued)

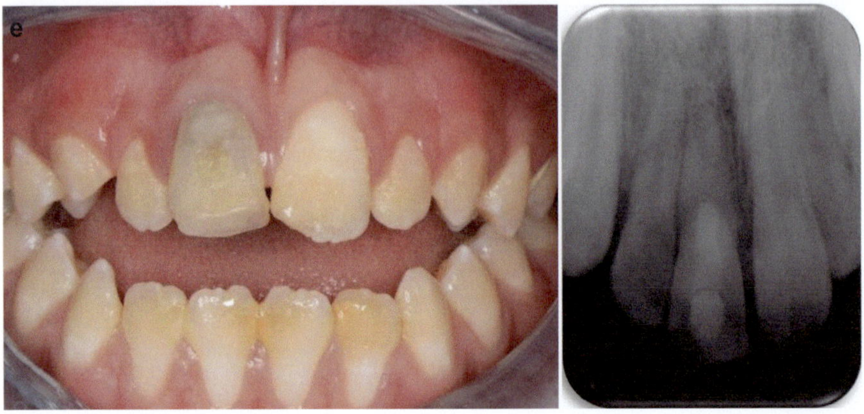

Fig. 8.7 (continued)

teeth with open apices are necessary to enable the entrance of blood vessels and stem cells into the canal space. The crown should be restorable without the need of a post in the canal space and the patient should be compliant [2].

Informed Consent

Informed consent must be obtained and signed by the patients' guardians. They should be informed that this procedure is relatively new with no accepted guidelines and that more than one visit is required. When intracanal antibiotic mix is used for disinfection the patient should be inquired about allergies and these antibiotics should be avoided. The patient should also be informed about possible tooth discoloration when antibiotic mix and/or MTA (even white) is used in the cervical area (Fig. 8.7d, e) [27, 28, 77]. Other treatment modalities for immature teeth with open apices (apexification, no treatment, or extraction) should be presented to the patient [2].

8.5.2.2 First Appointment

The tooth is anesthetized and isolated with a rubber dam. Straight line access opening is made to allow effective approach to the canal space for disinfection.

Disinfection of the Root Canal Space

Effective removal of necrotic pulp tissue and disinfection of the root canal are mandatory for any revascularization or regenerative endodontic response. The majority of studies report the use of irrigation combined with an intracanal medicament [2]. When choosing these disinfection agents a balance between the need to eliminate infection with the will to maintain the presence of vital stem cells should be considered. Surviving perivascular stem cells found in niches located in the apical papilla appears to be one origin of these cells [78, 79]. These stem cells are needed in order to populate the new scaffold created in the root canal space and under favorable conditions to migrate, proliferate and differentiate into functional pulp cells. The presence of HERS, which can survive traumatic events, allows continues development of root length.

The canal should be gently irrigated with NaOCl (20 mL/canal, 5 min) using an irrigation system that minimizes the possibility of extrusion of irrigants into the periapical space. Lower concentrations of NaOCl are recommended (1.5 %) and the irrigation needle is positioned about 3 mm from the root end, to minimize cytotoxicity to stem cells in the apical tissues. No mechanical debridement of the canal space is recommended [3, 60]. The canal is then irrigated with saline or 17 % EDTA (20 mL/canal, 5 min) and dried with paper points.

Two acceptable medicaments can be introduced into the canal space:

1. Low concentration of mixed antibiotic paste:
   The antibiotic combination of ciprofloxacin, metronidazole, and minocycline called Triple Antibiotic Paste (TAP) was introduced by Hoshino et al in 1996 [80]. It is prepared by mixing equal doses of the antibiotics with sterile saline to a paste-like consistency [2] and has been shown to be effective in eradicating bacteria *in vitro* [80, 81] and *in vivo* [82]. High concentration of TAP has a cytotoxic effect on stem cells, therefore a low concentration (0.1 mg/ml) is recommended [83, 84]. One of TAP's disadvantages is tooth greyish-green discoloration caused by minocycline (Fig. 8.7d, e) [77]. In order to avoid this discoloration eliminating minocycline is possible, replacing it with cefaclor [85] or using only two antibiotics [60]. Sealing the coronal dentin with composite and delivering TAP into the canal system with a syringe, in a back fill motion, can also help eliminate discoloration [86].
2. Calcium hydroxide:
   Calcium hydroxide is a strong antimicrobial agent and can dissolve necrotic tissue remnants in the canal [45–47]. Aqueous calcium hydroxide paste is placed only into the coronal half of the root canal via syringe in order to minimize its potential toxicity to vital stem cells [75].

   The access cavity is sealed with 3–4 mm of a temporary restorative material (i.e., Cavit- 3M, St. Paul, MN, USA or glass ionomer).

8.5.2.3 Second Appointment (2–4 Weeks After 1st Appointment)

First, an assessment of the initial treatment is done. Consistent symptoms and/or signs of infection requires additional treatment with the same medicament or a different one. The tooth is anesthetized with 3 % mepivacaine without vasoconstrictor, to allow bleeding into the canal space when it is mechanically induced, and isolated with a rubber dam. Irrigation with NaOCl is not recommended because of its cytotoxicity to stem cells and its ability to inhibit their adherence to dentin [2]. The canal is then irrigated gently with 17 % EDTA (20 ml/canal). Dentin conditioning with EDTA exposes collagen fibers on the dentin surface which may help the adhesion of new cells. It also releases bound growth factors that can attract new cells and promote their differentiation into odontoblast-like cells [66, 87]. After irrigation the canal is dried with paper points.

Scaffold

The apical tissue is agitated by over-instrumentation (endo file, endo explorer) to create a blood clot in the canal space ~3 mm below the cemento-enamel junction. Bleeding is stopped at this level with a cotton pellet soaked with sterile saline. It takes about 15 min for a stable blood clot to establish [75]. This blood clot provides a scaffold through which cells and a vasculature can grow [62, 65, 88] as well as a source of stem cells and factors that stimulate their growth and differentiation into odontoblast-like cells [78, 79]. Different materials have been proposed as alternatives to the creation of a blood clot i.e., platelet-rich plasma (PRP) [89], autologous fibrin matrix (AFM) [90], and collagen [91]. These alternatives should be further investigated.

MTA is placed over the blood clot to the level of the CEJ and acts as a pulp space barrier (Fig. 8.7b). Placing a resorbable matrix (such as CollaPlug- Zimmer Dental, Carlsbad, CA, USA) over the blood clot has been suggested in order to prevent the overextension of the MTA [92]. The use of gray and even white MTA has been associated with tooth discoloration [27, 28]. Therefore, in teeth where there is an esthetic concern alternatives to MTA (such as glass ionomer or Biodentine™ Allington Maidstone, Kent ME16 OJZ UK) should be considered [90]. It is important to note that the MTA placed in the cervical area prevents the maturation of the root in this prone-to-fracture spot and its influence is not clear [3].

After placement of the pulp space barrier, the final restoration is placed.

8.5.2.4 Follow Up

Follow up should consist of clinical and radiographic examinations. Clinical examination should reveal no pain, soft tissue swelling or sinus tract. Radiographic examination should reveal resolution of apical radiolucency and an increase in root length and wall thickness [2, 76].

The exact nature of the new tissue in the canal space is not clear. Radiographic evidence of changes in root length and wall thickness do not necessarily indicate a regeneration of functional pulp tissue and the formation of new dentin and cementum. Histologic studies in dogs and humans suggests that in some cases these radiographic changes may be a result of deposition of cementum-like and bone-like tissues, meaning, an ingrowth of periodontal ligament tissue instead of pulp tissue (Fig. 8.7c–e) [70, 74, 88, 93].

Considering the lack of clarity and predictability regarding the outcomes of procedures for pulpal regeneration to this day, some studies suggest that more information is needed before it can be routinely recommended [94, 95]. Some even suggest using it only as a last resort [96, 97].

8.6 Nonvital Pulp Treatment (Root Canal Treatment) for Young Mature Teeth

8.6.1 Special Considerations

Root canal treatment in mature teeth of children and adolescents is basically similar to that performed in adults. However, due to their wide canals and thin dentin walls in comparison with those of adult patients, special precautions are needed [1].

8.6.1.1 Access Opening

The coronal access should be wide enough to include the pulp horns to prevent future contamination and discoloration. During opening of the access cavity care should be taken to remove only a minimal amount of dentin in the canal orifices. Removing too much dentin will weaken anterior teeth and may cause perforation in molars.

8.6.1.2 Instrumentation

The length of the root canal should be determined carefully using radiographs. An electronic apex locator can also be used. Though the root canals are larger, they may be curved, so instrumentation should be done with precurved instruments in anti-curvature filing motions. The use of nickel titanium (NiTi) rotatory instruments will ease the preparation of the root canal.

8.6.1.3 Irrigation

Irrigation during root canal treatment should be done only after making sure that the rubber dam is placed properly, and that leakage of fluids into the mouth cannot occur accidentally. The needle of the irrigation syringe is placed loosely in the root canal to avoid pushing the irrigation solution beyond the apex. Sodium hypochlorite in various concentrations (0.5–5.25 %) is the preferred irrigation solution [50].

8.6.1.4 Intracanal Dressing

In teeth with infected root canals, the emphasis is on disinfection and removal of tissue remnants. Because effective mechanical preparation of wide canal walls is difficult, it is recommended that treatment be done in two appointments, with placement of an antiseptic dressing between visits. Calcium hydroxide is the preferred dressing material as it is antimicrobial and dissolves tissue remnants [45–47]. The placement of the dressing material can be done using a Lentulo spiral shorter than the length of the root canal, specially designed syringes or files.

8.6.1.5 The Isthmus

The isthmus is a thin communication between two or more root canals in the same root that contains pulp tissue. Any root containing more than one canal has a high incidence of isthmi [98]. An isthmus is formed when a root projection cannot close, and it will be larger in children where root formation is not fully complete. These web-like connections between root canals are part of the root canal system. They can function as a reservoir for bacteria and therefore should be cleaned and obturated during root canal treatment.

8.6.1.6 Obturation

The apical foramen in young teeth is large therefore adaptation of a master cone should be done carefully to avoid extrusion of filling materials that can easily occur during obturation. Lateral condensation requires more accessory gutta-percha points; initial points should be placed so that they will not block access to the canal. Filling with warm gutta-percha or use of warm condensation techniques should be done cautiously to avoid over extension.

In some cases fabrication of a customized master cone is favorable. A gutta-percha point is fitted several millimeters short of the apex, the apical 2–3 mm are softened (with a solvent or a heat source) and tamped gradually into place. The completed customized cone represents an impression of the apical portion of the canal preventing extrusion of filling material during obturation.

References

1. Fuks AB, Heling I, Nuni E. Pulp therapy for the young permanent dentition. In: Casamassimo PS, Fields HW, McTigue DJ, Nowak AJ, editors. Pediatric dentistry: infancy through adolescence. 5th ed. St. Louis: Saunders; 2013.
2. Law AS. Considerations for regeneration procedures. J Endod. 2013;39(3 Suppl):S44–56.
3. Cvek M. Prognosis of luxated non-vital maxillary incisors treated with calcium hydroxide and filled with gutta-percha. A retrospective clinical study. Endod Dent Traumatol. 1992;8(2):45–55.
4. Graham L, Cooper PR, Cassidy N, Nor JE, Sloan AJ, Smith AJ. The effect of calcium hydroxide on solubilisation of bio-active dentine matrix components. Biomaterials. 2006;27(14):2865–73.
5. Massagué J. The transforming growth factor-beta family. Annu Rev Cell Biol. 1990;6:597–641.
6. Mass E, Zilberman U, Fuks AB. Partial pulpotomy: another treatment option for cariously exposed permanent molars. ASDC J Dent Child. 1995;62(5):342–5.
7. Fuss Z, Trowbridge H, Bender IB, Rickoff B, Sorin S. Assessment of reliability of electrical and thermal pulp testing agents. J Endod. 1986;12(7):301–5.
8. Fulling HJ, Andreasen JO. Influence of maturation status and tooth type of permanent teeth upon electrometric and thermal pulp testing. Scand J Dent Res. 1976;84(5):286–90.
9. Johnsen DC, Harshbarger J, Rymer HD. Quantitative assessment of neural development in human premolars. Anat Rec. 1983;205:421–9.
10. Perez R, Berkowitz R, McIlveen L, Forrester D. Dental trauma in children: a survey. Endod Dent Traumatol. 1991;7(5):212–3.
11. AAE Consensus Conference Recommended Diagnostic Terminology. J Endod. 2009;35:1634.
12. AAE and AAOMR Joint Position Statement: use of cone beam computed tomography in endodontics 2015 update. Http://www.aae.org/uploadedfiles/clinical_resources/guidlines_and_position_statments/cbctstatement_2015update.pdf.
13. American Academy of Pediatric Dentistry: Guideline on pulp therapy for primary and immature permanent teeth, Revised 2014. Pediatric dentistry. Reference Manual 2014–2015; p. 242–50.
14. Schwendicke F, Dorfer C, Paris S. Incomplete caries removal: a systematic review and meta-analysis. J Dent Res. 2013;92(4):306–14.
15. Thompson V, Craig RG, Curro FA, Green WS, Ship JA. Treatment of deep carious lesions by complete excavation or partial removal: a critical review. J Am Dent Assoc. 2008;139(6):705–12.
16. Ricketts D, Lamont T, Innes NP, Kidd E, Clarkson JE. Operative caries management in adults and children. Cochrane Database Syst Rev. 2013;3:CD003808.
17. Ricketts DN, Kidd EA, Innes N, Clarkson J. Complete or ultraconservative removal of decayed tissue in unfilled teeth. Cochrane Database Syst Rev. 2006;(3):CD003808.
18. Cvek M. Endodontic management and the use of calcium hydroxide in traumatized permanent teeth. In: Andreasen JO, Andreasen FM, Andersson L, editors. Textbook and color atlas of traumatic injuries to the teeth. 4th ed. Oxford/Ames: Blackwell; 2007.
19. Bergenholtz G. Effect of bacterial products on inflammatory reactions in the dental pulp. Scand J Dent Res. 1977;85(2):122–9.
20. Bergenholtz G. Inflammatory response of the dental pulp to bacterial irritation. J Endod. 1981;7(3):100–4.
21. Parirokh M, Torabinejad M. Mineral trioxide aggregate: a comprehensive literature review-part I: chemical, physical, and antibacterial properties. J Endod. 2010;36(1):16–27.
22. Tronstad L, Andreasen JO, Hasselgren G, Kristerson L, Riis I. pH changes in dental tissues after root canal filling with calcium hydroxide. J Endod. 1981;7(1):17–21.

23. Witherspoon DE. Vital pulp therapy with new materials: new directions and treatment perspectives-permanent teeth. Pediatr Dent. 2008;30(3):220–4.
24. Schröder U. Effects of calcium hydroxide-containing pulp-capping agents on pulp cell migration, proliferation, and differentiation. J Dent Res. 1985;64:541–8.
25. Tziafas D, Smith AJ, Lesot H. Designing new treatment strategies in vital pulp therapy. J Dent. 2000;28(2):77–92.
26. Tziafas D, Pantelidou O, Alvanou A, Belibasakis G, Papadimitriou S. The dentinogenic effect of mineral trioxide aggregate (MTA) in short-term capping experiments. Int Endod J. 2002; 35(3):245–54.
27. Boutsioukis C, Noula G, Lambrianidis T. Ex vivo study of the efficiency of two techniques for the removal of mineral trioxide aggregate used as a root canal filling material. J Endod. 2008;34(10):1239–42.
28. Belobrov I, Parashos P. Treatment of tooth discoloration after the use of white mineral trioxide aggregate. J Endod. 2011;37(7):1017–20.
29. Vallés M, Mercadé M, Duran-Sindreu F, Bourdelande JL, Roig M. Influence of light and oxygen on the color stability of five calcium silicate-based materials. J Endod. 2013;39(4): 525–8.
30. Keskin C, Demiryurek EO, Ozyurek T. Color stabilities of calcium silicate-based materials in contact with different irrigation solutions. J Endod. 2015;41(3):409–11.
31. Akcay M, Sari S. The effect of sodium hypochlorite application on the success of calcium hydroxide and mineral trioxide aggregate pulpotomies in primary teeth. Pediatr Dent. 2014;36(4):316–21.
32. Schröder U. Effect of an extra-pulpal blood clot on healing following experimental pulpotomy and capping with calcium hydroxide. Odontol Revy. 1973;24(3):257–68.
33. Aguilar P, Linsuwanont P. Vital pulp therapy in vital permanent teeth with cariously exposed pulp: a systematic review. J Endod. 2011;37(5):581–7.
34. Mente J, Geletneky B, Ohle M, Koch MJ, Friedrich Ding PG, Wolff D, Dreyhaupt J, Martin N, Staehle HJ, Pfefferle T. Mineral trioxide aggregate or calcium hydroxide direct pulp capping: an analysis of the clinical treatment outcome. J Endod. 2010;36(5):806–13.
35. Qudeimat MA, Barrieshi-Nusair KM, Owais AI. Calcium hydroxide vs mineral trioxide aggregates for partial pulpotomy of permanent molars with deep caries. Eur Arch Paediatr Dent. 2007;8(2):99–104.
36. Cvek M. A clinical report on partial pulpotomy and capping with calcium hydroxide in permanent incisors with complicated crown fracture. J Endod. 1978;4(8):232–7.
37. Cvek M, Cleaton-Jones PE, Austin JC, Andreasen JO. Pulp reaction to exposure after experimental crown fractures or grinding in adult monkeys. J Endod. 1982;8(9):391–7.
38. Granath LE, Hagman G. Experimental pulpotomy in human bicuspids with reference to cutting technique. Acta Odontol Scand. 1971;29(2):155–63.
39. Tziafas D, Molyvdas I. The tissue reactions after capping of dog teeth with calcium hydroxide experimentally crammed into the pulp space. Oral Surg Oral Med Oral Pathol. 1988;65(5): 604–8.
40. Oginni AO, Adekoya-Sofowora CA, Kolawole KA. Evaluation of radiographs, clinical signs and symptoms associated with pulp canal obliteration: an aid to treatment decision. Dent Traumatol. 2009;25(6):620–5.
41. Heide S, Kerekes K. Delayed partial pulpotomy in permanent incisors of monkeys. Int Endod J. 1987;20(2):65–74.
42. Kaiser HJ. Management of wide open apex canals with calcium hydroxide. Presented at the 21st annual meeting of the American Association of Endodontists, Washington DC 17 Apr 1964.
43. Sheehy EC, Roberts GJ. Use of calcium hydroxide for apical barrier formation and healing in non-vital immature permanent teeth: a review. Br Dent J. 1997;183(7):241–6.
44. Rafter M. Apexification: a review. Dent Traumatol. 2005;21(1):1–8.
45. Hasselgren G, Olsson B, Cvek M. Effects of calcium hydroxide and sodium hypochlorite on the dissolution of necrotic porcine muscle tissue. J Endod. 1988;14(3):125–7.

46. Kim D, Kim E. Antimicrobial effect of calcium hydroxide as an intracanal medicament in root canal treatment: a literature review- part I. In vitro studies. Restor Dent Endod. 2014;39(4):241–52.
47. Kim D, Kim E. Antimicrobial effect of calcium hydroxide as an intracanal medicament in root canal treatment: a literature review- part II. In vivo studies. Restor Dent Endod. 2015;40(2):97–103.
48. Andreasen JO, Farik B, Munksgaard EC. Long-term calcium hydroxide as a root canal dressing may increase risk of root fracture. Dent Traumatol. 2002;18(3):134–7.
49. Hatibović-Kofman S, Raimundo L, Zheng L, Chong L, Friedman M, Andreasen JO. Fracture resistance and histological findings of immature teeth treated with mineral trioxide aggregate. Dent Traumatol. 2008;24(3):272–6.
50. Mohammadi Z. Sodium hypochlorite in endodontics: an update review. Int Dent J. 2008;58(6): 329–41.
51. van der Sluis LW, Versluis M, Wu MK, Wesselink PR. Passive ultrasonic irrigation of the root canal: a review of the literature. Int Endod J. 2007;40(6):415–26.
52. Metzger Z, Solomonov M, Mass E. Calcium hydroxide retention in wide root canals with flaring apices. Dent Traumatol. 2001;17(2):86–92.
53. Seghi RR, Nasrin S, Draney J, Katsube N. Root fortification. J Endod. 2013;39(3 Suppl):S57–62.
54. Giuliani V, Baccetti T, Pace R, Pagavino G. The use of MTA in teeth with necrotic pulps and open apices. Dent Traumatol. 2002;18(4):217–21.
55. Abouqal R, Rida S. Apexification of immature teeth with calcium hydroxide or mineral trioxide aggregate: systematic review and meta-analysis. Oral Surg Oral Med Oral Pathol Oral Radiol Endod. 2011;112(4):e36–42.
56. Lee YL, Lee BS, Lin FH, Yun Lin A, Lan WH, Lin CP. Effects of physiological environments on the hydration behavior of mineral trioxide aggregate. Biomaterials. 2004;25(5):787–93.
57. Yeung P, Liewehr FR, Moon PC. A quantitative comparison of the fill density of MTA produced by two placement techniques. J Endod. 2006;32(5):456–9.
58. Trope M. Treatment of immature teeth with non-vital pulps and apical periodontitis. Dent Clin North Am. 2006;54(2):313–24.
59. Patino MG, Neiders ME, Andreana S, Noble B, Cohen RE. Collagen as an implantable material in medicine and dentistry. J Oral Implantol. 2002;28(5):220–5.
60. Iwaya SI, Ikawa M, Kubota M. Revascularization of an immature permanent tooth with apical periodontitis and sinus tract. Dent Traumatol. 2001;17(4):185–7.
61. Banchs F, Trope M. Revascularization of immature permanent teeth with apical periodontitis: new treatment protocol? J Endod. 2004;30(4):196–200.
62. Kling M, Cvek M, Mejare I. Rate and predictability of pulp revascularization in therapeutically reimplanted permanent incisors. Endod Dent Traumatol. 1986;2(3):83–9.
63. Andreasen JO, Borum MK, Jacobsen HL, Andreasen FM. Replantation of 400 avulsed permanent incisors. 1. Diagnosis of healing complications. Endod Dent Traumatol. 1995;11(2):59–68.
64. Claus I, Laureys W, Cornelissen R, Dermaut LR. Histologic analysis of pulpal revascularization of autotransplanted immature teeth after removal of the original pulp tissue. Am J Orthod Dentofacial Orthop. 2004;125(1):93–9.
65. Skoglund A, Tronstad L. Pulpal changes in replanted and autotransplanted immature teeth of dogs. J Endod. 1981;7(7):309–16.
66. Murray PE, Garcia-Godoy F, Hargreaves KM. Regenerative endodontics: a review of current status and a call for action. J Endod. 2007;33(4):377–90.
67. Nygaard-Ostby B. The role of the blood clot in endodontic therapy: an experimental histologic study. Acta Odontol Scand. 1961;19:323–53.
68. Nygaard-Ostby B, Hjortdal O. Tissue formation in the root canal following pulp removal. Scand J Dent Res. 1971;79(5):333–49.
69. Horsted P, Nygaard-Ostby B. Tissue formation in the root canal after total pulpectomy and partial root filling. Oral Surg Oral Med Oral Pathol. 1978;46(2):275–82.
70. Wang X, Thibodeau B, Trope M, Lin LM, Huang GT. Histologic characterization of regenerated tissues in canal space after the revitalization/revascularization of immature dog teeth with apical periodontitis. J Endod. 2010;36(1):56–63.

71. Huang GT, Lin LM. Letter to the editor: comments on the use of the term "revascularization" to describe root regeneration. J Endod. 2008;34(5):511.
72. Hargreaves KM, Giesler T, Henry M, Wang Y. Regeneration potential of the young permanent tooth: what does the future hold? J Endod. 2008;34(7 Suppl):S51–6.
73. Trope M. Reply. J Endod. 2008;34:511–2.
74. Huang GT. Apexification: the beginning of its end. Int Endod J. 2009;42(10):855–66.
75. Wigler R, Kaufman AY, Lin S, Steinbock N, Hazan-Molina H, Torneck CD. Revascularization: a treatment for permanent teeth with necrotic pulp and incomplete root development. J Endod. 2013;39(3):319–26.
76. American Association of Endodontists. Considerations for regenerative procedures. Available at: http://www.aae.org/clinical-resources/regenerative-endodontics/considerations-for-regenerative-procedures.aspx. Revised 12 Apr 2015.
77. Kim JH, Kim Y, Shin SJ, Park JW, Jung IY. Tooth discoloration of immature permanent incisor associated with triple antibiotic therapy: a case report. J Endod. 2010;36(6):1086–91.
78. Huang GT, Sonoyama W, Liu Y, Liu H, Wang S, Shi S. The hidden treasure in apical papilla: the potential role in pulp/dentin regeneration and bioroot engineering. J Endod. 2008;34(6): 645–51.
79. Lovelace TW, Henry MA, Hargreaves KM, Diogenes A. Evaluation of the delivery of mesenchymal stem cells into the root canal space of necrotic immature teeth after clinical regenerative endodontic procedure. J Endod. 2011;37(2):133–8.
80. Hoshino E, Kurihara-Ando N, Sato I, Uematsu H, Sato M, Kota K, Iwaku M. In-vitro antibacterial susceptibility of bacteria taken from infected root dentine to a mixture of ciprofloxacin, metronidazole and minocycline. Int Endod J. 1996;29(2):125–30.
81. Sato I, Ando-Kurihara N, Kota K, Iwaku M, Hoshino E. Sterilization of infected root-canal dentine by topical application of a mixture of ciprofloxacin, metronidazole and minocycline in situ. Int Endod J. 1996;29(2):118–24.
82. Windley W, Teixeira F, Levin L, Sigurdsson A, Trope M. Disinfection of immature teeth with a triple antibiotic paste. J Endod. 2005;31(6):439–43.
83. Chuensombat S, Khemaleelakul S, Chattipakorn S, Srisuwan T. Cytotoxic effects and antibacterial efficacy of a 3-antibiotic combination: an in vitro study. J Endod. 2013;39(6):813–9.
84. Ruparel NB, Teixeira FB, Ferraz CC, Diogenes A. Direct effect of intracanal medicaments on survival of stem cells of the apical papilla. J Endod. 2012;38(10):1372–5.
85. Thibodeau B, Trope M. Pulp revascularization of a necrotic infected immature permanent tooth: case report and review of the literature. Pediatr Dent. 2007;29(1):47–50.
86. Reynolds K, Johnson JD, Cohenca N. Pulp revascularization of necrotic bilateral bicuspids using a modified novel technique to eliminate potential coronal discolouration: a case report. Int Endod J. 2009;42(1):84–92.
87. Galler KM, D'Souza RN, Federlin M, Cavender AC, Hartgerink JD, Hecker S, Schmalz G. Dentin conditioning codetermines cell fate in regenerative endodontics. J Endod. 2011;37(11):1536–41.
88. Thibodeau B, Teixeira F, Yamauchi M, Caplan DJ, Trope M. Pulp revascularization of immature dog teeth with apical periodontitis. J Endod. 2007;33(6):680–9.
89. Iwaya S, Ikawa M, Kubota M. Revascularization of an immature permanent tooth with periradicular abscess after luxation. Dent Traumatol. 2011;27(1):55–8.
90. Geisler TM. Clinical considerations for regenerative endodontics procedures. Dent Clin North Am. 2012;56(3):603–26.
91. Yamauchi N, Yamauchi S, Nagaoka H, Duggan D, Zhong S, Lee SM, Teixeira FB, Yamauchi M. Tissue engineering strategies for immature teeth with apical periodontitis. J Endod. 2011;37(3):390–7.
92. Petrino JA, Boda KK, Shambarger S, Bowles WR, McClanahan SB. Challenges in regenerative endodontics: a case series. J Endod. 2010;36(3):536–41.
93. Becerra P, Ricucci D, Loghin S, Gibbs JL, Lin LM. Histologic study of a human immature permanent premolar with chronic apical abscess after revascularization/revitalization. J Endod. 2014;40(1):133–9.

94. Andreasen JO, Bakland LK. Pulp regeneration after non-infected and infected necrosis, what type of tissue do we want? A review. Dent Traumatol. 2012;28(1):13–8.
95. Alobaid AS, Cortes LM, Lo J, Nguyen TT, Albert J, Abu-Melha AS, Lin LM, Gibbs JL. Radiographic and clinical outcomes of the treatment of immature permanent teeth by revascularization or apexification: a pilot retrospective cohort study. J Endod. 2014;40(8):1063–70.
96. Garcia-Godoy F, Murray PE. Recommendations for using regenerative endodontic procedures in permanent immature traumatized teeth. Dent Traumatol. 2012;28(1):33–41.
97. Slutzky-Goldberg I, Heling I. Revascularization? Only as the last resort! Refuat Hapeh Vehashinayim. 2013;30(3):30–5, 62.
98. Estrela C, Rabelo LE, de Souza JB, Alencar AH, Estrela CR, Sousa Neto MD, Pécora JD. Frequency of root canal isthmi in human permanent teeth determined by cone-beam computed tomography. J Endod. 2015;41(9):1535–9.

The Future: Stem Cells and Biological Approaches for Pulp Regeneration

9

Jacques E. Nör and Carolina Cucco

Contents

9.1 Introduction

Achieving long-lasting and complete pulp regeneration in teeth with deep caries or severe trauma remains a significant clinical challenge. In teeth with immature apices and exposed vital pulp tissue, partial or complete pulpotomy is typically indicated to preserve pulp function and allow for continued root development. In cases

J.E. Nör, DDS, MS, PhD (✉)
Department of Cariology, Restorative Sciences, Endodontics, University of Michigan School of Dentistry, 1011 N University Rm. 2353, Ann Arbor, MI 48109-1078, USA
e-mail: jenor@umich.edu

C. Cucco, DDS, MS, PhD
Department of Cariology, Restorative Sciences, Endodontics, University of Michigan School of Dentistry, 1011 N University Rm. 2310G, Ann Arbor, MI 48109-1078, USA
e-mail: cuccocarolina@gmail.com

A.B. Fuks, B. Peretz (eds.), *Pediatric Endodontics: Current Concepts in Pulp Therapy for Primary and Young Permanent Teeth*,
DOI 10.1007/978-3-319-27553-6_9

where injury caused loss of pulp vitality and arrested root development, teeth may remain with poor crown-to-root ratio, a root with very thin walls, and an open apex. The ideal treatment in such cases would be to regenerate a functional dentin–pulp complex that would enable the completion of root development and thickening of dentinal walls. Emerging evidence suggests that this can be achieved with the recruitment of apical stem cells toward the root canal and/or the transplantation of stem cells using a tissue engineering-based approach. In this chapter, we will discuss the evidence that provides the rationale for regenerative approaches for the treatment of pulp injury or pulp necrosis.

Conservative pulp therapies have been used for many years in an attempt to maintain pulp vitality in teeth with injury. However, with the discovery of the function of stem cells in dental pulp tissue, the search for biological approaches that exploit these cells for pulp regeneration has intensified exponentially. It is well known that the dental pulp is vulnerable to insults, such as caries, infection, and trauma. Whereas current approaches for treatment of these conditions focus primarily on the maintenance of the compromised tooth structure, future approaches have as ultimate goal the complete regeneration of dental tissues (i.e., dentin and pulp), even in cases of pulp necrosis in young teeth [1, 2]. With the emphasis on tissue regeneration and tooth viability, these new concepts of regenerative endodontic procedures aim at enhancing the strength of the tooth and sustain (or recover) pulp vitality [1–3].

With the isolation of postnatal stem cells from various sources in the oral cavity and the development of biocompatible materials for cell and growth factor delivery, possibilities for alternative, cell biology-based treatments are becoming more feasible. Interdisciplinary approaches will be needed to move from replacement to regeneration, involving clinicians as well as cell biologists and material scientists. In this chapter, we will first discuss basic principles of tooth development, which can be applied to recreate signaling events to inspire dental tissue engineering approaches. For the regeneration of individual tooth structures, the classical tissue engineering triad, i.e., stem cells, scaffold materials, and morphogenic factors [4], is discussed. New tissue engineering initiatives focused on the regeneration of the dentin–pulp complex will be presented. In projecting future directions, we conclude with a brief discussion of key components necessary to develop effective strategies for dental pulp tissue engineering, which might enable us to implement novel regenerative strategies in clinical practice in the near future.

9.2 Pulp Therapy in Primary and Young Permanent Teeth

In recent years, there has been an increasing focus on conservative strategies in endodontics for the treatment of diseased dental pulps. Within the emerging paradigm of regenerative endodontics, stem cell and tissue engineering technologies offer potential for repair and regeneration of dentin–pulp tissues in the treatment of necrotic teeth [1, 2]. Dental pulp was identified 10 years ago as an accessible tissue from which to isolate postnatal mesenchymal stem cells, especially from exfoliating primary teeth, premolars, and permanent molars extracted for orthodontic reasons.

These cells constitute an excellent stem cell source for dental tissue regeneration, owing to their high accessibility, proliferative ability, and multilineage differentiation potential [5, 6].

During development, odontogenesis progresses through molecular cross talk and reciprocal interactions between two morphologically different tissues, the ectoderm and the underlying mesenchyme [5]. This characteristic developmental pattern was found to be a key mechanism orchestrating the morphogenesis of other systems including hair and glands [6]. Understanding the underlying molecular mechanisms of tooth formation is key to enable recreation of these processes for dental tissue engineering purposes. A unique set of signaling molecules, including sonic hedgehog and bone morphogenetic proteins, play critical roles in the control tooth patterning [7]. During tooth development, the shifting interactions between epithelium and mesenchyme depend on the developmental stage (see Chap. 2). Understanding the temporal and spatial patterns of these interactions might be a key factor in recapitulating the developmental profile of tooth formation to engineer dental tissues in the future.

9.3 Regeneration of the Dental Pulp

The regeneration of individual tooth structures is a more realistic approach in the short term, as compared to regeneration of the entire tooth. The first primary cultures of stem cells derived from adult dental pulp were named dental pulp stem cells (DPSCs) [8]. Soon after that, exfoliated deciduous teeth were also identified as an important source of postnatal stem cells (stem cells from human exfoliated deciduous teeth, SHED) [9]. Both DPSC and SHED are clonogenic, form adherent cell clusters, and are capable of multilineage differentiation [8–11]. Compared with bone marrow stromal stem cells, they show 30–50 % higher proliferation rates and increased population doublings [9]. Microarray analysis revealed distinct gene expression patterns for DPSC compared with bone marrow stromal stem cells [12]. Expression of mineralization markers and formation of mineralized nodules are observed when these cells are cultured in the presence of inductive media containing ascorbic acid, dexamethasone, and inorganic phosphate [8, 9, 13–15]. After transplantation in vivo, both DPSC and SHED are able to regenerate dentin–pulp-like complexes, as those shown in Fig. 9.1 [16–19]. Banking and storage services for cells from exfoliated primary teeth or extracted permanent teeth are becoming widely available throughout the world.

Pulp-related stem cells can also be harvested from dental papilla, the organ that generates the dental pulp during tooth development. These stem cells from apical papilla, which give rise to the odontoblasts that are responsible for root dentin formation, can be harvested from developing wisdom teeth, and they show a high capacity for dentin regeneration, as they are likely to be less differentiated compared with DPSCs [20, 21].

Tooth-derived mesenchymal stem cells express STRO-1, a putative mesenchymal stem cell marker; their potential to differentiate into odontoblasts, osteoblasts, adipocytes, and neural cells has been demonstrated [8–10, 13, 15, 22]. DPSCs were

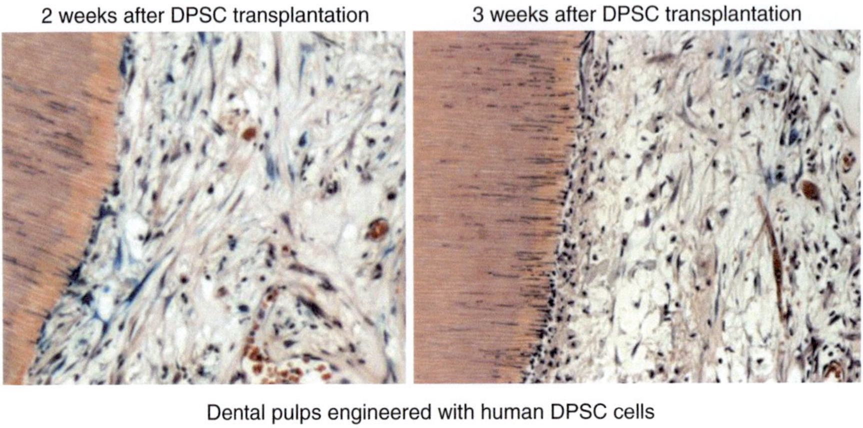

Fig. 9.1 Human dental pulps engineered with human dental pulp stem cells (DPSCs). Postnatal stem cells (DPSCs) were seeded in tooth slice/scaffolds and transplanted into the subcutaneous space of immunodeficient mice. Photomicrographs of engineered pulps 2 or 3 weeks after transplantation. To identify the human DPSCs, we stably transduced them with the LacZ gene that makes these cells blue in response to staining with β-galactosidase

also shown to be positive for alpha-smooth muscle actin, CD146, and pericyte-associated antigen (3G5) [12]. Notably, it was recently demonstrated that dental pulp stem cells reside in perivascular niches [23].

9.4 Growth and Differentiation Factors

Enhanced understanding of the biological processes involved in both tooth development and repair are creating conditions to enhance reparative responses and tissue regeneration. The dentin matrix contains innumerous proteins and growth factors capable of stimulating tissue repair. These growth factors are secreted by pulp cells and deposited within the dentin matrix during mineralization [24, 25] where they remain protected in active forms. Demineralization of the dentin after application of cavity-etching agents or dressing for pulp capping [26], or even during cavity preparation [27, 28], releases these growth factors and makes them available to the surrounding cells. They seem to play key roles in controlling many of the events of reparative dentin formation [10, 29]. Growth factors, especially those of the transforming growth factor (TGF)-beta family, are important players in cellular signaling; they stimulate odontoblast differentiation and dentin matrix secretion, leading to increased reparative dentin formation [29].

Another important family of growth factors in tooth development and regeneration are the bone morphogenetic proteins (BMP). Recombinant human BMP-2 stimulates the differentiation of adult pulp stem cells into an odontoblast-like cell type in culture [30, 31]. Similar inductive effects of TGF-beta 1–3 and BMP-7 have been demonstrated in cultured tooth slices [32, 33]. Recombinant BMP-2, BMP-4, and BMP-7 induce formation of reparative dentin in vivo [30, 34]. The application of recombinant human insulin growth factor (IGF)-1 has been found to induce dentin bridging, comparable to a calcium hydroxide-based capping agent [35]. In addition to growth factors, other molecules have been shown to stimulate pulp cell differentiation. Dentin matrix protein (DMP)-1, a noncollagenous protein involved in mineralization processes, induces cytodifferentiation, collagen synthesis, and calcified deposits after direct pulp capping in animal models [36]. Dexamethasone, a synthetic glucocorticoid, reduces cell proliferation and induces expression of alkaline phosphatase and dentin sialophosphoprotein in primary human dental pulp cells [37]. The addition of beta-glycerophosphate to the cell culture medium in explants from human teeth induced a change in cell morphology, collagen synthesis, and mineral formation [38]. Combinations of dexamethasone with inorganic phosphate have been used for dental stem cell differentiation and the induction of mineralization in several studies [8, 9]. The key message here is that there are known biological regulators of dental pulp cell behavior that have been considered as potentially viable therapeutic strategies for regenerative endodontic procedures.

9.5 Scaffolds

Scaffolds are carriers for cells, which provide a 3D environment for cell adhesion, migration, and differentiation. Ideally, they should biodegrade at the same rate as the new tissues form. Scaffold materials should be biocompatible and nontoxic. For dental pulp tissue engineering, the injectable materials are advantageous. Natural polymers, such as collagen, elastin, glycosaminoglycans, fibrin, alginate, silk, and chitosan, have long been used as carriers [39]. Although these materials provide structural strength and are biocompatible and biodegradable, they offer few possibilities for controlling the structure or making compositional modifications to improve their performance. Synthetic polymers, on the other hand, provide high control of the mechanical and chemical properties. Polylactic acid (PLA), polyglycolic acid (PGA), and their copolymer poly(lactic-co-glycolic acid) (PLGA) have been widely used for tissue engineering applications including regenerative dentistry [40, 41]. Hydrogel is particularly interesting because of their tissue-like viscoelastic properties, efficient transport of nutrients and metabolic products, uniform cell encapsulation, and the possibility of injection and gelation in situ. Gels have been made from polyethylene glycol fibrin, glycosaminoglycans, or peptide-based building blocks. Based on their chemistry, they can be chemically or physically cross-linked, and modifications such as the incorporation of biofunctional molecules or growth and differentiation factors are possible [42].

9.6 Tissue Engineering in Endodontics

The concept of tissue engineering was conceived by Langer and Vacanti in the early 1990s to describe the technique for biological tissue regeneration [43]. Tissue engineering refers to the science of generating new living tissues to replace, repair, or augment the diseased/damaged tissue and restore tissue/organ function [44].

The objectives of tissue engineering procedures in endodontics are to regenerate a pulp-like tissue and ideally the pulp–dentin complex. An immature tooth with a necrotic pulp does not have residual progenitor pulpal cells to continue root development [45–47]. The main goals of conventional root canal therapy, including complete cleaning and shaping and appropriate obturation, cannot be achieved in an immature root. Moreover, the short, weak, and fracture-prone root of an immature tooth [48] becomes even weaker after mechanical instrumentation of the root canal. Apexification with $Ca(OH)_2$ [49] or an apical plug [50] may solve many of the problems associated with conventional root canal therapy; however, there is still the risk of horizontal root fracture especially at the cervical area and tooth mobility due to compromised crown-to-root ratio (Chap. 8).

Apexification with $Ca(OH)_2$ was proposed by Frank (1966), in which $Ca(OH)_2$ is used in multiple visits during a long period of treatment to induce an apical barrier [49]. In addition to the extended treatment period, long-term contact of dentin with $Ca(OH)_2$ decreases the mechanical strength of dentin, making the tooth susceptible to fracture [51, 52]. Cvek (1992) reported a higher incidence of cervical root fracture in root-filled immature teeth compared to mature teeth following dental trauma [48]. Therefore, preserving (or restoring) the pulp vitality of immature teeth with deep caries or dental trauma is of great importance.

To keep the tooth vital, several research groups are pursuing the idea of engineering dental pulp, which was initially proposed by David Mooney's group at the University of Michigan in the nineties [53, 54]. Dental pulp fibroblasts were cultured on PGA scaffolds for 60 days, and the cells were proliferated and formed tissue similar to native dental pulp [53]. Bohl et al. tested whether different scaffold materials influenced the proliferation and collagen synthesis of dental pulp fibroblasts 2 years later and found PGA to be the most conducive compared with alginate and collagen type I hydrogel [54]. A dental pulp-like tissue was generated using DPSCs in combination with collagen scaffolds and DMP-1 as a morphogenic factor on dentin slices after transplantation in vivo [55]. Our group used SHED cells seeded onto polymer scaffolds within tooth slices and transplanted these constructs into immunocompromised mice. A pulp-like tissue formed within the tooth slices after 2–4 weeks, the cells lining the dentin showed expression of odontoblast/osteoblast markers, and microvessel formation was observed [16]. Notably, SHED differentiated into odontoblasts that synthesized new tubular dentin, confirming their differentiation into fully functional odontoblastic cells [17].

Galler's group demonstrated the growth and differentiation of stem cells derived from different dental tissues in a PEGylated fibrin hydrogel. The cells degraded the fibrin, replaced it with a collagenous matrix, and deposited mineral after osteogenic induction. Furthermore, SHED and DPSCs were tested for compatibility with a self-assembling peptide hydrogel, which offers several possibilities to modify the matrix. The optimization of a peptide sequence through the incorporation of the cell adhesion motif RGD (arginine–glycine–aspartic acid) and a matrix metalloproteinase (MMP)-2-specific enzyme cleavable site led to increased proliferation rates and enhanced migration of SHED and DPSCs into these matrices [56]. Furthermore, studies with peptide-based hydrogels showed that the differentiation of dental pulp stem cells can be stimulated in this type of matrix [57]. Further steps toward a tailor-made system include the incorporation and slow release of growth and differentiation factors, such as TGF-beta1, FGF2, and VEGF.

9.7 Approaches for Regenerative Endodontics

The following are possible approaches (Fig. 9.2) that have been explored for dental pulp tissue regeneration: (A) root canal revascularization via blood clotting, (B) postnatal stem cell transplantation using injectable scaffolds, and (C) pulp transplantation using stem cells grown in sheets. These techniques are based on the basic tissue engineering principles and include specific consideration of stem cells, growth factors, and scaffolds. Of these approaches, the only one that is currently approved for general clinical use in the USA and in several other countries throughout the world is the "root canal revascularization via blood clotting" procedure, as called simply "revascularization" (see Chap. 8). Nevertheless, the approaches employing stem cell transplantation are areas of intense basic and translational research that should lead to clinical transplantation in the not so distant future.

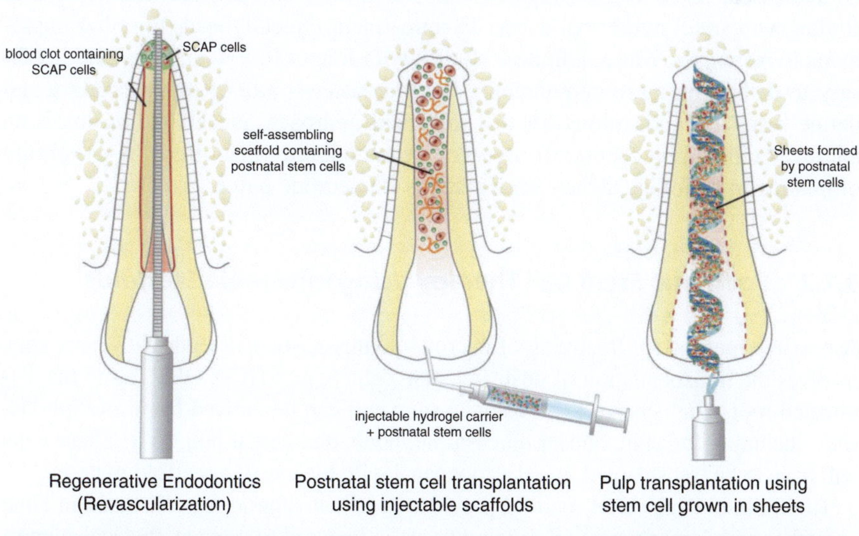

Fig. 9.2 Current strategies for the engineering of dental pulps. Diagram depicting three strategies for the engineering of human dental pulps, as follows: (**a**) root canal revascularization via blood clotting, (**b**) postnatal stem cell transplantation using injectable scaffolds, and (**c**) pulp transplantation using stem cells grown in sheets

9.7.1 Root Canal "Revascularization" via Blood Clotting

Nygaard Ötsby (1961) first described the concept of revascularization, indicating sustained root development following blood clot induction in the root canal of immature teeth suffering from pulp necrosis. Accordingly, the ideal outcome for teeth with an immature root and necrotic pulp would be formation of vascularized tissue in the canal space capable of inducing normal root development [58, 59].

The regeneration process depends on the presence of osteoblast and odontoblast progenitor stem cells in the apical dental papilla, which might be resistant to infection and necrosis within the canal due to their vicinity to periodontal blood vessels [60]. The aim is to create a suitable environment so that the periapical stem cells can proliferate into the root canal space for regeneration of pulp tissue and continuation of root development [61].

This technique involves the instrumentation of the root canal beyond the apex with the objective of forming a blood clot. It involves the use of intracanal irrigants (e.g., diluted sodium hypochlorite, chlorhexidine) with placement of antibiotics (a mixture of ciprofloxacin, metronidazole, and minocycline paste) for several weeks. This particular combination of antibiotics effectively disinfects the root canal system and increases revascularization of the necrotic tooth [62, 63]. This approach is being increasingly used as it is relatively simple and can be completed using standard instruments and medicaments. Notably, the regeneration of tissue in root canal systems occurs by a patient's own blood cells avoiding the possibility of immune rejection or pathogen transmission from replacing the pulp with a tissue-engineered construct.

Despite the simple technique of revascularization, several concerns still need to be addressed. Most of the support for this technique comes from case reports or studies with small number of cases. This treatment typically leads to rather unpredictable responses. More definitive studies with longer follow-up times are necessary to determine more convincingly the true success rate of this procedure and define better the indications for this treatment approach. Nevertheless, this is an approved clinical procedure for regenerative endodontics that offers the possibility of treating in a biological way young teeth with necrotic pulps.

9.7.2 Postnatal Stem Cell Therapy Using Injectable Scaffolds

A possible method for treatment of necrotic young permanent teeth with open apex involves the transplantation of postnatal stem cells (e.g., SHED, DPSC) into the disinfected root canal system [3]. Postnatal stem cell can be derived from multiple tissues, including the skin, buccal mucosa, fat, bone, and dental pulp [64]. These cells will have to be transplanted into the root canal with the use of a scaffold material.

Rigid tissue-engineered scaffold provides excellent support for cells used in bone and other body areas where engineered tissue is required to provide physical support [65]. However, in root canal system, a tissue-engineered pulp is not required to provide structural support of the tooth. This will allow tissue-engineered pulp tissue to be administered in a soft 3D scaffold matrix such as hydrogel. Hydrogel is an injectable scaffold that can be delivered by syringe [66]. The hydrogel has the potential to be noninvasive and easy to deliver into the root canal system. It promotes pulp regeneration by providing a substrate for cell proliferation and differentiation into an organized tissue structure [67]. To make hydrogel more practical, research is focusing on making them photopolymerizable to form rigid structures once they are implanted into the tissue site. Work from the Galler laboratory [68] is focused on the development of functionalized injectable scaffolds that can be used for regenerative endodontic approaches. Indeed, this is a very exciting area of research and a tremendous opportunity for collaborations between clinicians, material scientists, and cell biologists.

We have shown that the implantation of SHED cells into full roots of premolars transplanted in the subcutaneous of immunodeficient mice results in the regeneration of functional dental pulps throughout the extent of the root canal [69]. This was particularly successful when we used PuraMatrix as an injectable scaffold for cell delivery. In contrast, transplantation of SHED cells in recombinant human collagen type I matrices was not as successful, as demonstrated by the presence of areas of odontoclastic activity. Ongoing clinical trials conducted by Dr. Misako Nakashima and colleagues in Japan are beginning to explore the safety and efficacy of postnatal stem cell transplantation for the treatment of necrotic permanent teeth.

9.7.3 Pulp Transplantation Using Stem Cells Grown in Sheets

In this case, replacement pulp tissue is generated in vitro and then transplanted into a clean root canal of a necrotic tooth. The cellular source for the replacement pulp tissue could be cells taken from a biopsy or an exfoliated primary tooth that has been expanded in the laboratory. The cultured pulp tissue is grown in sheets in vitro on biodegradable polymer nanofibers or in a sheet of extracellular matrix protein such as collagen I or fibronectin [70]. These sheets of pulp-like tissue would then be rolled to form a cylinder that can be implanted into the disinfected root canal. These sheets are not very difficult to grow and are likely more stable than an injection of dissociated cells. However, sheets of cells lack vascularity, and therefore the apical portion of the canal has the highest likelihood to be conducive to the survival of the cells in these constructs [71]. Another potential challenge is the fact that these cellular sheets are extremely fragile, making it difficult to place them in the root canal without breakage. Hence, this approach still needs to be further optimized prior to consideration for clinical use. Notably, the Sfeir group recently demonstrated that dental pulp stem cells in 3D self-assembled scaffoldless sheets can be used to regenerate a vital pulp-like tissue in tooth root canal systems. These recent data suggest a promising new method to deliver stem cells into root canals for pulp regeneration therapies [72].

Conclusions

Contemporary dentistry relies heavily on biomaterials to replace lost tissues in the oral cavity. Such strategies restore shape and form, but do not necessarily regenerate the physiological architecture and function of the lost tissue. However, advances in the field of material sciences, stem cell biology, and dental tissue engineering have raised the possibility of using biology-based treatment strategies that are fundamentally developed to regenerate functional dental tissues. Proof-of-concept studies have demonstrated the possibility of generating complete teeth. However, there are formidable challenges that will have to be overcome before complete tooth replacement becomes a clinical reality, including reproducing the size, shape, and color of natural teeth. On the other hand, the regeneration of a specific dental tissue at the time appears to be more feasible in the short run. It is particularly exciting to see the exponential development in the field of dental pulp tissue regeneration. The development of a clinically feasible approach that results in a safe, cost-effective, and consistently efficacious strategy for dental pulp tissue regeneration will require the work of multidisciplinary teams consisted of clinicians, material scientists, and cell biologists.

References

1. Petersen PE. World Health Organization global policy for improvement of oral health – World Health Assembly 2007. Int Dent J. 2008;58(3):115–21.
2. Casagrande L, Cordeiro MM, Nör SA, Nör JE. Dental pulp stem cells in regenerative dentistry. Odontology. 2011;99(1):1–7.
3. Nör JE. Tooth regeneration in operative dentistry. Oper Dent. 2006;31(6):633–42.
4. Nakashima M, Reddi AH. The application of bone morphogenetic proteins to dental tissue engineering. Nat Biotechnol. 2003;21(9):1025–32.
5. Thesleff I. Epithelial-mesenchymal signaling regulating tooth morphogenesis. J Cell Sci. 2003;116(Pt 9):1647–8.
6. Pispa J, Thesleff I. Mechanisms of ectodermal organogenesis. Dev Biol. 2003;262(2):195–205.
7. Thesleff I, Mikkola M. The role of growth factors in tooth development. Int Rev Cytol. 2002;217:93–135.
8. Gronthos S, Mankani M, Brahim J, Robey PG, Shi S. Postnatal human dental pulp stem cells (DPSCs) in vitro and in vivo. Proc Natl Acad Sci U S A. 2000;97(25):13625–30.
9. Miura M, Gronthos S, Zhao M, et al. SHED: stem cells from human exfoliated deciduous teeth. Proc Natl Acad Sci U S A. 2003;100(10):5807–12.
10. Gronthos S, Brahim J, Li W, et al. Stem cell properties of human dental pulp stem cells. J Dent Res. 2002;81(8):531–5.
11. Paino F, Ricci G, De Rosa A, et al. Ecto-mesenchymal stem cells from dental pulp are committed to differentiate into active melanocytes. Eur Cell Mater. 2010;20:295–305.
12. Shi S, Robey PG, Gronthos S. Comparison of human dental pulp and bone marrow stromal stem cells by cDNA microarray analysis. Bone. 2001;29:532–9.
13. Seo BM, Miura M, Gronthos S, et al. Investigation of multipotent postnatal stem cells from human periodontal ligament. Lancet. 2004;364(9429):149–55.
14. Wei X, Ling J, Wu L, Liu L, Xiao Y. Expression of mineralization markers in dental pulp cells. J Endod. 2007;33(6):703–8.
15. Gay IC, Chen S, MacDougall M. Isolation and characterization of multipotent human periodontal ligament stem cells. Orthod Craniofac Res. 2007;10(3):149–60.
16. Cordeiro MM, Dong Z, Kaneko T, et al. Dental pulp tissue engineering with stem cells from exfoliated deciduous teeth. J Endod. 2008;34(8):962–9.
17. Sakai VT, Zhang Z, Dong Z, et al. SHED differentiate into functional odontoblasts and endothelium. J Dent Res. 2010;89(8):791–6.
18. Demarco FF, Casagrande L, Zhang Z, Dong Z, Tarquino SB, Zeitlin BD, Shi S, Smith AJ, Nör JE. Effects of morphogen and scaffold porogen on the differentiation of dental pulp stem cells. J Endod. 2010;36(11):1805–11.

19. Sonoyama W, Liu Y, Yamaza T, et al. Characterization of the apical papilla and its residing stem cells from human immature permanent teeth: a pilot study. J Endod. 2008;34(2):166–71.
20. Huang GT, Sonoyama W, Liu Y, Liu H, Wang S, Shi S. The hidden treasure in apical papilla: the potential role in pulp/dentin regeneration and bioroot engineering. J Endod. 2008;34:645–51.
21. Iohara K, Nakashima M, Ito M, Ishikawa M, Nakasima A, Akamine A. Dentin regeneration by dental pulp stem cell therapy with recombinant human bone morphogenetic protein 2. J Dent Res. 2004;83(8):590–5.
22. Machado CV, Passos ST, Campos TM, Bernardi L, Vilas-Bôas DS, Nör JE, Telles PD, Nascimento IL. The dental pulp stem cell niche based on aldehyde dehydrogenase 1 expression. Int End J. 2015. doi:10.1111/iej.12511. [Epub ahead of print].
23. Smith AJ, Matthews JB, Hall RC. Transforming growth-factor-b1 (TGF-b1) in dentin matrix. Ligand activation and receptor expression. Eur J Oral Sci. 1998;106 Suppl 1:179–84.
24. Roberts-Clark DJ, Smith AJ. Angiogenic growth factors in human dentine matrix. Arch Oral Biol. 2000;45(11):1013–6.
25. Smith AJ, Cassidy N, Perry H, Begue-Kirn C, Ruch JV, Lesot H. Reactionary dentinogenesis. Int J Dev Biol. 1995;39:273–80.
26. Graham L, Cooper PR, Cassidy N, Nör EJ, Sloan AJ, Smith AJ. The effect of calcium hydroxide on solubilization of bio-active dentine matrix components. Biomaterials. 2006;27(14):2865–73.
27. Murray PE, Smith AJ. Saving pulps – a biological basis. An overview. Prim Dent Care. 2002;9(1):21–6.
28. Tziafas D. Basic mechanisms of cytodifferentiation and dentinogenesis during dental pulp repair. Int J Dev Biol. 1995;39:281–90.
29. Tziafas D, Alvanou A, Panagiotakopoulos N. Induction of odontoblast-like cell differentiation in dog dental pulps after in vivo implantation of dentine matrix components. Arch Oral Biol. 1995;40(10):883–93.
30. Smith AJ, Murray PE, Sloan AJ, Matthews JB, Zhao S. Trans-dentinal stimulation of tertiary dentinogenesis. Adv Dent Res. 2001;15:51–4.
31. Nakashima M, Nagasawa H, Yamada Y, Reddi AH. Regulatory role of transforming growth factor-b, bone morphogenetic protein-2, and protein-4 on gene expression of extracellular matrix proteins and differentiation of dental pulp cells. Dev Biol. 1994;162(1):18–28.
32. Iohara K, Zheng L, Ito M, Tomokiyo A, Matsushita K, Nakashima M. Side population cells isolated from porcine dental pulp tissue with self-renewal and multipotency for dentinogenesis, chondrogenesis, adipogenesis, and neurogenesis. Stem Cells. 2006;24(11):2493–503.
33. Sloan AJ, Smith AJ. Stimulation of the dentine–pulp complex of rat incisor teeth by transforming growth factor-b isoforms 1–3 in vitro. Arch Oral Biol. 1999;44(2):149–56.
34. Sloan AJ, Rutherford RB, Smith AJ. Stimulation of the rat dentine–pulp complex by bone morphogenetic protein-7 in vitro. Arch Oral Biol. 2000;45(2):173–7.
35. Six N, Decup F, Lasfargues JJ, Salih E, Goldberg M. Osteogenic proteins (bone sialoprotein and bone morphogenetic protein-7) and dental pulp mineralization. J Mater Sci Mater Med. 2002;13(2):225–32.
36. Lovschall H, Fejerskov O, Flyvberg A. 63 pulp-capping with recombinant human insulin-like growth factor I (rhIGF-I) in rat molars. Adv Dent Res. 2001;15:108–12.
37. Almushayt A, Narayanan K, Zaki AE, George A. Dentin matrix protein 1 induces cytodifferentiation of dental pulp stem cells into odontoblasts. Gene Ther. 2006;13(7):611–20.
38. Alliot-Licht B, Bluteau G, Magne D, et al. Dexamethasone stimulates differentiation of odontoblast-like cells in human dental pulp cultures. Cell Tissue Res. 2005;321(3):391–400.
39. Couble ML, Farges JC, Bleicher F, Perrat Mabillon B, Boudeulle M, Magloire H. Odontoblast differentiation of human dental pulp cells in explant cultures. Calcif Tissue Int. 2000;66(2):129–38.
40. Gomes A, Azevedo H, Malafaya P, et al. Tissue engineering, van Blitterswijk C, editor. Burlington/San Diego: Elsevier; 2008.

41. Chan G, Mooney DJ. New materials for tissue engineering: towards greater control over the biological response. Trends Biotechnol. 2008;26(7):382–92.
42. Langer R, Tirrell DA. Designing materials for biology and medicine. Nature. 2004; 428(6982):487–92.
43. Langer R, Vacanti JP. Tissue engineering. Science. 1993;260(5110):920–6.
44. Curtis M, Riehle M. Tissue engineering: the biophysical background. Phys Med Biol. 2001;46(4):47–65.
45. Torneck CD, Smith J. Biologic effects of endodontic procedures on developing incisor teeth. I. Effect of partial and total pulp removal. Oral Surg Oral Med Oral Pathol. 1970;30:258–66.
46. Torneck CD, Smith JS, Grindall P. Biologic effects of endodontic procedures on developing incisor teeth. II. Effect of pulp injury and oral contamination. Oral Surg Oral Med Oral Pathol. 1973;35:378–88.
47. Torneck CD, Smith JS, Grindall P. Biologic effects of endodontic procedures on developing incisor teeth. 3. Effect of debridement and disinfection procedures in the treatment of experimentally induced pulp and periapical disease. Oral Surg Oral Med Oral Pathol. 1973; 35:532–40.
48. Cvek M. Prognosis of luxated non-vital maxillary incisors treated with calcium hydroxide and filled with gutta-percha. A retrospective clinical study. Endod Dent Traumatol. 1992;8:45–55.
49. Frank AL. Therapy for the divergent pulpless tooth by continued apical formation. J Am Dent Assoc. 1966;72:87–93.
50. Torabinejad M, Chivian N. Clinical applications of mineral trioxide aggregate. J Endod. 1999;25:197–205.
51. Kleier CJ, Barr ES. A study of endodontically apexified teeth. Endod Dent Traumatol. 1991;7:112–7.
52. Mohammadi Z, Dummer PM. Properties and applications of calcium hydroxide in endodontics and dental traumatology. Int Endod J. 2011;44:697–730.
53. Mooney DJ, Powell C, Piana J, Rutherford B. Engineering dental pulp-like tissue in vitro. Biotechnol Prog. 1996;12(6):865–8.
54. Bohl KS, Shon J, Rutherford B, Mooney DJ. Role of synthetic extracellular matrix in development of engineered dental pulp. J Biomater Sci Polym. 1998;9(7):749–64.
55. Prescott RS, Alsanea R, Fayad MI, et al. In vivo generation of dental pulp-like tissue by using dental pulp stem cells, a collagen scaffold, and dentin matrix protein 1 after subcutaneous transplantation in mice. J Endod. 2008;34(4):421–6.
56. Galler KM, Aulisa L, Regan KR, D'Souza RN, Hartgerink JD. Self-assembling multidomain peptide hydrogels: designed susceptibility to enzymatic cleavage allows enhanced cell migration and spreading. J Am Chem Soc. 2010;132(9):3217–23.
57. Galler KM, Cavender A, Yuwono V, et al. Self-assembling peptide amphiphile nanofibers as a scaffold for dental stem cells. Tissue Eng Part A. 2008;14(12):2051–8.
58. Ötsby BN. The role of the blood clot in endodontic therapy. An experimental histologic study. Acta Odontol Scand. 1961;19:324–53.
59. Torabinejad M, Turman M. Revitalization of tooth with necrotic pulp and open apex by using platelet-rich plasma: a case report. J Endod. 2011;37:265–8.
60. Whitherspoon DE, Small JC, Regan JD, Nunn M. Retrospective analysis of open apex teeth obturated with mineral trioxide aggregate. J Endod. 2008;34:1171–6.
61. Hargreaves KM, Giesler T, Henry M, Wang Y. Regeneration potential of the young permanent tooth: what does the future hold? J Endod. 2008;37(7 suppl):S51–6.
62. Sato I, Ando-Kurihara N, Kota K, Iwaku M, Hoshino E. Sterilization of infected root-canal dentine by topical application of a mixture of ciprofloxacin, metronidazole and minocycline in situ. Int Endod J. 1996;29:118–24.
63. Hoshino E, Kurihara-Ando N, Sato I, et al. In-vitro antibacterial susceptibility of bacteria taken from infected root dentine to a mixture of ciprofloxacin, metronidazole and minocycline. Int Endod J. 1996;29:125–30.
64. Kindler V. Postnatal stem cell survival: does the niche, a rare harbor where to resist the ebb tide of differentiation, also provide lineage-specific instructions? J Leukoc Biol. 2005;78:836–44.

65. Trojani C, Weiss P, Michiels JF, et al. Three-dimensional culture and differentiation of human osteogenic cells in an injectable hydroxypropyl-methylcellulose hydrogel. Biomaterials. 2005;26:5509–17.
66. Alhadlaq A, Mao JJ. Tissue-engineered osteochondral constructs in the shape of an articular condyle. J Bone Joint Surg Am. 2005;87:936–44.
67. Luo Y, Shoichet MS. A photolabile hydrogel for guided three-dimensional cell growth and migration. Nat Mater. 2004;3:249–53.
68. Galler KM, Cavender AC, Koeklue U, Suggs LJ, Schmalz G, D'Souza RN. Bioengineering of dental stem cells in PEGylated fibrin gel. Regen Med. 2011;6(2):191–200.
69. Rosa V, Zhang Z, Grande RH, Nör JE. Dental pulp tissue engineering in full length human root canals. J Dent Res. 2013;92(11):970–5.
70. Venugopal J, Ramakrishna S. Applications of polymer nanofibers in biomedicine and biotechnology. Appl Biochem Biotechnol. 2005;125:147–58.
71. Peter SJ, Miller MJ, Yasko AW, Yaszemski MJ, Mikos AG. Polymer concepts in tissue engineering. J Biomed Mater Res. 1998;43:422–7.
72. Syed-Picard FN, Ray Jr HL, Kumta PN, Sfeir C. Scaffoldless tissue-engineered dental pulp cell constructs for endodontic therapy. J Dent Res. 2014;93(3):250–5.

Index

A.B. Fuks, B. Peretz (eds.), *Pediatric Endodontics: Current Concepts in Pulp Therapy for Primary and Young Permanent Teeth*,
DOI 10.1007/978-3-319-27553-6